SILENT HUNGER

Dedicated to all
Thin Within Graduates

*This special edition is an expression
of our sincere appreciation
for your unique contribution
to our quest for the truth.
This book is a tribute
to your struggles as well as your victories.
Without you it could not have been written.*

*In his name
Judy and Arthur
Summer 1994*

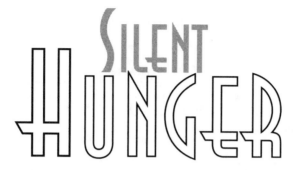

SILENT HUNGER

*A Biblical Approach
to Overcoming Compulsive Eating
and Overweight*

Arthur W. Halliday, M.D.
Judy Wardell Halliday, R.N.

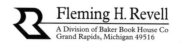

Fleming H. Revell
A Division of Baker Book House Co
Grand Rapids, Michigan 49516

Published by Fleming H. Revell
a division of Baker Book House Company
P.O. Box 6287, Grand Rapids, MI 49516-6287

Printed in the United States of America

Library of Congress Cataloging-in-Publication Data

Halliday, Arthur

    Silent hunger / Arthur and Judy Halliday.
    p. cm.
    ISBN 0-8007-5524-3
    1. Compulsive eaters—Religious aspects—Christianity. 2. Relationship addiction—Religious aspects—Christianity. 3. Reducing—Religious aspects—Christianity. 4. Interpersonal relations—Religious aspects—Christianity. 5. Obesity—Religious aspects—Christianity. I. Halliday, Judy Wardell II. Title.
BV4596.C58H35   1994
261.8'3225—dc20   93-33904

Hearken to the sound of my cry . . .

Psalm 5:2

This book is affectionately dedicated
to all our counselees
who have honored us with their trust
and taught us much of what we know
about God's miraculous healing
and
to Mom and Dad Wardell
who have been a constant source
of steadfast love

Contents

Acknowledgments

We gratefully acknowledge these people who have contributed significantly to this book:

- The thousands of Thin Within graduates who have shared their struggles as well as their victories and who have taught us far more than we have taught them.
- All of our faithful friends who have prayed for us over these many years.
- The pastoral staff of Peninsula Bible Church—Brian Morgan, Gary Vanderet, and John Hanneman—for their excellent teaching of the Scriptures.
- Serena O'Farrell, our dear friend, who patiently and prayerfully persevered with us in the writing of this book.
- Sheila Kogan Flannery, our treasured friend, whose helpful suggestions brought clarity to this manuscript.
- Pat Patmore and Jane Alexander for their wisdom, support, and suggestions.
- Special thanks to Roy M. Carlisle, our agent, for all of his support and encouragement during the years of discussions and planning involved in the birthing process of this book.
- Heartfelt gratitude to Joy Imboden Overstreet, cofounder of Thin Within and special friend since 1975, whose contribution made this book possible.
- Sincere appreciation to Linda Wilder for the many hours she spent reading the manuscript, making invaluable suggestions, and openly sharing the joys and sorrows of her life.

- Bill Petersen, our publisher, for his belief in this message, his faith in us, and his expertise in the publishing process.
- David Eckman, Executive Dean, Western Seminary, for teaching us about our love and acceptance in Jesus Christ.
- Debra Sands Miller, our collaborator, who spent hundreds of hours organizing our material and presenting it in a lucid literary form. For all of your effort and for being courageous when the going was tough, our deep gratitude.
- Most importantly we give thanks and all praise to our Lord and Savior. We hope and pray that this message is consistent with your Word and that it will minister to many of your flock.

Introduction

Hunger is a universal experience. Television, newspapers, and magazines bring wide-eyed and sunken-cheeked faces from around the world into our homes and our hearts, and we are grieved. Yet even those of us fortunate enough to have an abundance of food are hungry. We sit down three times a day to tables laden with food, but our deepest hunger is not satisfied.

Each of us has a hunger deep within where no one can see. And although it may not be obvious, this hunger is the most universal of all. It is the silent hunger of the starving soul. It is silent because we don't recognize it or have words to describe it; silent because it has been muted with years of behavior designed to still its voice; silent because the noise of our world prevents it from being heard.

But this hunger cannot be completely silenced. It cries out to be heard. It is our compelling desire to be loved, protected, and considered precious. It is a God-given hunger for genuine intimacy wherein our deepest needs for security and significance can be substantially met.

Unfortunately, when these needs are not met, we turn to counterfeits such as food, drugs, alcohol, work, or other compulsions in an attempt to fill the void. But if the bad news is that our attempts to satisfy this hunger on our own have failed, the good news is that God has provided the means to eternal fulfillment, satisfaction, and a life of freedom. You may wonder how this is possible, but the Scriptures tell us: "With man this is impossible, but with God all things are possible" (Matt. 19:26).

11

God's way is the way of faith and freedom. When we bring our struggles with food, eating, and weight to him in honest surrender, we can be restored. For this to happen we must allow God to lead us to a place where we are:

- Free to risk—letting go of the past in order to live unencumbered in the present (1 Peter 5:6–7)
- Free to change—being transformed from the inside out by the renewing of our minds (Rom. 12:2)
- Free to trust—trusting God and the way he made us (1 Cor. 6:19)
- Free to love—loving as Christ loves us (John 13:34)

As we act in faith and surrender to this kind of freedom, we will experience a new relationship with God, with ourselves, and with our bodies. We will be able to:

- Eat in response to our true, physiological hunger
- Stop eating when we are satisfied
- Eat the foods we enjoy and which nourish and satisfy us

We present the principles for this kind of eating in this book. These principles are not rigid rules or fixed formulas; they are God-centered principles that respect the way God created our bodies. They are designed to preserve our freedom.

As you read this book, you will hear the stories of men and women who have experienced this freedom for themselves as they discovered and resolved the issues that lay beneath their struggles with food, eating, and weight. Their testimonies, as well as those of countless others who have graciously shared with us during the past thirty-five years of medical practice and nineteen years of Thin Within workshops and counseling sessions, demonstrate the profound courage it takes to face whatever prevents us from listening to the voice of our silent hunger.

At some point we must acknowledge that *food is not the problem.* While this book is written primarily for those whose struggles concern food, it is also for those who have attempted to bury their inner needs under layers of habitual behaviors of any kind. It is our hope and prayer that you will discover that *your silent hunger can be satisfied*—with the true bread of life, our living God.

If you are willing to listen to the voice of your silent hunger, you will find that God is present to soothe, satisfy, and make you feel secure in ways that nothing of this world can. And as he satisfies your silent hunger, you will find that, miraculously, your struggles will cease to be the focus of your life. As you are restored, you will regain your dignity in relationship to yourself, others, and God. As you grow to know, appreciate, and love the body God created uniquely for you, you will come to see yourself as he sees you—the wondrous and deeply beloved child of God that you are. And you will find your security and significance in him.

Hunger is the doorway through which God enters our soul. He takes this place of greatest vulnerability and weakness and uses it to restore, satisfy, and sanctify us. And in the profound silence that accompanies his presence we hear him say, "Blessed are you who hunger now, for you will be satisfied" (Luke 6:21).

Part 1

Free
to Risk

1

Intimacy Not Counterfeits

"Are you thirsty?" said the Lion.
"I'm dying of thirst," said Jill.
"Then drink," said the Lion.
"May I—could I—would you mind going away while I
    do?" said Jill.
The Lion answered this only by a look and a very low
    growl. . . .
"I daren't come and drink," said Jill.
"Then you will die of thirst," said the Lion.
"Oh dear!" said Jill, coming a step nearer. "I suppose I must
    go and look for another stream then."
"There is no other stream," said the Lion.

C. S. Lewis
The Silver Chair

Have you been searching for a stream of refreshment that will
satisfy the yearning of your soul? We are a people consumed with
an insatiable thirst or hunger for something we cannot name,

something that will soothe and satisfy us, something that will give us a sense of peace. We sit down three times a day to tables laden with food, yet our deepest hunger is never satisfied. All too often, not knowing what is wrong or what will fulfill our longing, we turn to food, drugs, alcohol, sex, workaholism, or other counterfeits. When our eating is out of control or when food is used to insulate ourselves against emotional pain, we say that our eating is disordered, that it is out of God's order. Disordered eating is characterized as follows:

- Where we are preoccupied with concerns of food and eating.
- Where food is used to insulate or numb ourselves from emotional pain.
- Where food is used in an attempt to satisfy our unfulfilled yearnings to be loved, cherished, and adored.
- Where food or eating is used to try to achieve some order in a disordered life.
- Where the joy and pleasure of eating has been lost.
- Where food or eating has become a compulsion, an obsession, or an idol.
- Where food or eating causes a disruption in life.
- Where food and eating control us rather than vice versa.
- Where food has become an enemy rather than a friend.

Disordered eating becomes a counterfeit for genuine satisfaction and leaves us empty and longing.

What throws our natural, God-given ability to determine our hunger and satisfy it appropriately into such disorder? The following stories illustrate some of the circumstances that may disrupt the natural cycle of hunger and satisfaction and lead to disordered eating.

Denette's Story

My father was a successful farmer who traveled a great deal during the winter months, while my mother stayed home to raise my younger brother and me. My father was rather passive, whereas my mother was opinionated and controlling. She made all of my decisions for me and imposed on me her desire that I become a ballerina. I began dance lessons at age five, and my mother put me on my first diet when I was six. I'd get so hungry I would sneak food at my friends' houses, often eating a whole box of cookies or cereal at one time. Then I'd purge to keep the perfect body my mother insisted I have. When I was eleven years old, my parents divorced and my mother had to go to work to support the family.

---

*Disordered eating becomes
a counterfeit for genuine satisfaction and
leaves us empty and longing.*

Four years later my brother died suddenly, and my mother was devastated. He had clearly been her favorite, because of his high academic achievements. I felt she would have preferred that I had died, so I tried harder and harder to please her. I became a perfectionist—equating love with approval—but I was never able to live up to my mother's expectations. When I didn't act, feel, think, or dress to her standards, she would show her disapproval by withdrawing emotionally.

I left home for the first time when I went to college. On my way back to my dormitory one night, I was raped. When my mother found out about this by reading my diary, she warned me never to tell anyone about the shameful incident. I began to eat uncontrollably and gained fifty pounds.

I met my first boyfriend later that year, and soon we dated steadily. When he broke off the relationship, I was crushed and began to focus more on my body, convinced that if I could just lose weight, everything would be better. I saw one therapist after another in an effort to change my eating habits, but nothing helped. My drive to become thin increased until I was anorexic and bulimic.

Years later, after my mother's death from cancer, I participated in a Thin Within workshop. Only then did I begin to look at the pain and loss hidden beneath my eating disorder and to start the journey toward wholeness. The most significant outcome of the three years of counseling that followed was that I learned to place God at the center of my life. My eating is now normal, and I have learned to relate and express my feelings to my husband, my children, and in my friendships.

Alexis's Story

I was one of three attractive, intelligent, seemingly "perfect" daughters. My mother was quiet and passive; my father was a successful professional, who would not admit he had a drinking problem. He often flew into sudden, prolonged rages and bouts of verbal abuse that would leave me devastated and in tears. I never knew when these outbursts would occur or what prompted them.

When I was ten, my parents sent me to a boarding school where I was harshly criticized and severely punished if my performance was unsatisfactory. When I told my parents, they said I would just have to adjust and warned me *not* to make waves. I felt unprotected and vulnerable, and my feelings of self-worth gradually eroded.

When I was twenty-two, I married a man who had been abandoned at age five by his alcoholic father, and although he wanted to be a good companion, his own insecurities caused him to be critical and controlling. I tried to do everything to please him, since I considered him the "perfect one" in our marriage. After two children and little intimacy, I had a secret, extramarital affair and turned to food and alcohol to cope with my unhappiness and guilt. I was not significantly overweight, but I would frequently binge until my stomach hurt so badly I would have to lie down and sleep it off.

As my marriage deteriorated and my alcohol and food consumption increased, I began to verbally abuse my children. My rage got out of control, and at this point I sought Christian counseling. When I was asked to look at my past, I said, "Why? Things weren't so bad when I was growing up. I know of many families where things were much worse." It wasn't until I was able to articulate the abuse I experienced as a child and separate my earthly father from my heavenly Father—accepting a godly perspective of myself as a valuable and beloved person—that I began to change the way I related to my husband and children.

It took me two years of perseverance and prayer to see more clearly how I had used my eating behaviors to cope. I have chosen to abstain from alcohol, and I no longer binge eat. Facing the past and taking responsibility for the choices I make in the present have given me a new experience of freedom, both in my eating and in my relationships.

David's Story

I was one of ten siblings raised in a Christian home with an alcoholic father who embarrassed and abused us. We learned early on *not* to discuss our feelings.

I married when I was nineteen, and I worked hard to become a successful businessman. Because of arguments over sex, my marriage was stormy from the beginning. My inner rage became so intense that I would lose control, and in frustration I physically abused my wife. For the sake of appearances and our three children, we agreed to stay together but to sleep in separate bedrooms. I had several extramarital affairs during this time, for which I felt extremely guilty.

After fifteen years of an empty marriage, my wife was killed in an automobile accident in which I was the driver. This event was so painful that I began to eat compulsively to numb the memory and the feelings of intense guilt.

I went to my church for counsel but was told to rejoice that my wife was now with the Lord, to be strong, and not to cry. Unable to express my feelings and having no permission to grieve, I continued overeating until I was extremely obese. Food helped me suppress my sexual urges and bury my feelings of shame and guilt.

I tried countless weight-loss programs, including two visits to the Pritikin Institute. My physicians continually urged me to lose weight, and I would lose some for a time, only to gain it back and more. Eventually I developed severe coronary artery disease and underwent two bypass surgeries.

When I first began counseling for my disordered eating, I believed I had resolved the guilt and pain over my wife's death. When asked about it, I remarked with confidence, "I have grieved and put it all behind me." But suddenly the memory of my wife's death was so vivid, it was as if she had died yesterday, and I wept for the first time. The pain, shame, and guilt I experienced with that memory were so intense I knew I had finally broken through the wall of denial that kept me from grieving for years—and from forgiving myself and asking forgiveness from others as well as God.

I am 110 pounds lighter today but still in the process of healing. I have, with much prayer, begun to heal from the emotional abuse of my childhood. As I release the past pain, my weight continues to decrease. I stand on God's promise that he will complete the good work he has started in me.

Hannah's Story

I was an exuberant, expressive child born to a quiet, depressed mother and a father who didn't want to be married. They divorced when I was two. My mother grieved in silence, and my father never visited. I was alone with painful feelings, longings, and unanswered questions. That feeling of isolation remained with me for years. While I was an affectionate child, I learned very early that my mother was uncomfortable with her body and any physical displays of affection. So I kept my feelings and my emotions to myself. As I grew I yearned for a daddy like my friends had, but I had to be silent about it. How I felt about anything was clearly of no importance to my mother, so I turned to the most predictable comforters I knew—my dog and food.

When I was ten, some high school boys invited me to their attic hideout for an "initiation rite," which involved my touching them and them fondling me. When I told my mother, I was scolded and told that I should never speak of it again.

The years of high school, college, marriage, and motherhood did nothing to shift my perception of myself as deeply flawed and of my feelings as invalid on important issues. I continued to numb myself with food, my drug of choice, until I was quite overweight. Even becoming a Christian didn't give me much hope. I just felt guilty for being so out of control.

Thin Within jarred me into the truth of what I had to risk to change my life. I refused to face it at first, but as I stopped over-eating and started praying, I began to accept God's love and to know that he validates me just as I am. So far I have released over sixty pounds, but what is even more significant is that I feel *free*. By being willing to experience my hunger I became more open to the joy *and* the pain in my life. With God's help I am choosing to change old patterns, to trust myself, and to love and be loved.

Although each of the above experiences is unique, all reflect disordered eating as a response to emotional pain. None of these four people consciously chose to disrupt their natural cycle of eat-ing, and none understood when they came for help how their food, eating, and weight related to their past. Yet each has found the way to stop the cycle of disordered eating that disrupted their lives.

Can't You Just Stop?

How often have your parents, friends, spouse, or you yourself asked, "Don't you have any willpower?" "Why don't you just put down your fork and refuse a second helping!" "Why don't you just say no?"

When our eating is disordered, we may lament with the apos-tle Paul, "I do not understand what I do. For what I want to do I do not do, but what I hate I do" (Rom. 7:15). We often do not understand why we do what we hate to do with food. All we know is that nothing we have tried so far has helped us, and we are afraid we will never be able to change. We may assume, too, that we are somehow to blame for our weakness. This produces addi-tional shame and guilt, and we begin to label ourselves as hope-less, stupid, and worthless. But is this true?

The answer is a resounding no. Like Denette, Alexis, David, and Hannah, we have adopted patterns of disordered eating in an unconscious attempt to insulate ourselves against emotional pain.

How many of us can tell stories like these? Our pasts are marked with events and experiences that wounded our esteem, deprived us of security, and left us feeling insignificant and alone. We yearn for something that will permanently satisfy us. The irony is that we end up substituting a counterfeit—a disordered relationship with food, eating, and weight—for what can truly satisfy us.

Causes of Disordered Eating

Each of the four stories at the beginning of this chapter illustrates an experience or event that left the person hungering. At some point in each person's life, there was a breach, collapse, or lack of intimacy. Each adopted patterns of disordered eating in an unconscious attempt to insulate him- or herself against the emotional pain. The various causes of disordered eating, adapted from the *Eating Disorders* manual,[1] might be listed as follows:

1. *Trauma:* This includes any single event that causes unresolved emotional trauma. Specific examples might be the death of a close relative or friend, divorce, leaving home for the first time, rape, abortion, rejection in a significant relationship, emotional or physical abandonment, a traumatic sexual experience, or even a critical remark.
2. *Abuse:* Abuse is physical, verbal, sexual, or emotional assault. It may be short- or long-term and may be the result of an ongoing unresolved conflict, such as an unhappy or abusive marriage. Extended abuse might include growing up in a dysfunctional home situation (for example, with an alcoholic parent).
3. *Having been a very sensitive child:* Two children with different personality types, raised in the same environment, may respond and develop very differently. Even in a "functioning" family, where feelings are acknowledged, a very sensitive child may not have his or her needs met. A child who grows up in a family where emotional pain is not acknowledged or discussed may turn to food for comfort. Outwardly the family may appear to be "perfect" and problem-free. Frequently these families are very religious and spend a signif-

icant amount of time attending church or synagogue activities. Even though the source of the family's pain is often very subtle and difficult to identify, children are usually aware of it and maybe even think it is their fault. Lacking someone to talk to and having inadequate coping skills, a child may develop disordered eating.

4. *A controlling environment:* People who have grown up with a parent or have married a person who is very controlling may try to survive by giving up their own identities while trying to please the other people. If this becomes too painful or is no longer acceptable, a person may be unable to reestablish his or her own identity and may have difficulty making even simple decisions regarding food and eating.

5. *Lack of validation of feelings:* Many people with eating disorders come from families or relationships where there appears to be no overt abuse or identifiable problem. They experienced, rather, a very subtle undermining of their self-esteem, as did Hannah. They may have repeatedly received no validation of their thoughts or feelings or were given the message that it was wrong or selfish to feel as they did. People (as children or as adults) might conclude from this experience that they must be bad or crazy. Over time, they learned, as Hannah did, to direct their negative emotions inwardly and become self-abusive, since direct expression was not allowed.

The common thread in each of these situations is that the security and unconditional love necessary for healthy emotional growth and expression are not present. As a result, the emotional pain experienced could not be managed in a healthy way. Families of people who develop disordered eating "do not model intimacy or allow feelings to be expressed in a way that promotes closeness, support, or resolution of conflict."[2] Consequently, they do not develop the ability to ask for what they need. The result may be disordered eating, where one turns to food as a source of comfort, security, and love. One of our workshop participants said: "I started overeating when I was thirteen. As soon as I felt emotionally uncomfortable, I would eat. I used food for solace and comfort. Even when it no longer eased my pain, it had become such a habit that I couldn't break free." She finds that when she eats, the pain is buried or subdued.

Disordered eating can also result when you are "successful" in managing your weight. When you "lose" excess pounds, people make comments like, "Oh, you look so good! You've lost weight!" You may begin to feel acceptable, loved, and approved on that basis for the first time in your life. Where once life seemed painful and out of control, now there is something within your control that brings positive attention.[3] You may find that the more you focus on counting calories, exercising, dieting, losing weight, or purging, the less you feel the emotional pain. But always present within us is a hunger we realize isn't being satisfied. We are hungry, but what are we hungry for?

Silent Hunger

Our silent hunger is our longing for intimacy where our deepest needs for security and significance can be substantially met. This longing is real. It is a sanctified hunger placed in us by God's design, and it is his intention that it be satisfied in our families, with our friends, but most completely in communion with him.

Intimacy includes our need to love and be loved, to be valued and cherished, to be treated with dignity and respect, and to relate to one another at the deepest, most authentic level of our being. This need for intimacy can be met only in the context of intimate relationships. "The fabric of Biblical truth is woven from Genesis to Revelation with the thread of relationship."[4] In fact, God's plan for us is summed up in our intimate relationship with him— Immanuel, God with us. He intends our deepest need for intimacy to be met in *relationships,* heavenly and earthly.

Our need for intimacy—for connectedness and expression of our innermost character—is one of our most basic human needs. It is fundamental to our physical, mental, and spiritual health and to our ability to live the lives of self-giving love God intends for us. From it springs our ability to develop the elements necessary for the continued development of healthy relationships and normal coping behaviors in our lives. But in a fallen world our formative relationships are often broken or distorted, and intimacy is impaired or missing. Unsatisfied and unfulfilled, we ache with a silent hunger. To appease it we often develop compulsive behavior that results in food, eating, and weight becoming the focus of our lives.

> *Our need for intimacy—for connectedness and expression of our innermost character— is one of our most basic human needs.*

When we confuse the emotional and spiritual needs of our silent (soul) hunger with the nutritional needs of our physiological hunger, we may attempt to satisfy our need for intimacy and emotional satisfaction with disordered eating, a counterfeit relationship with food. We may end up binge eating, purging, or dieting excessively, focusing on how fat we are or how much we hate our bodies rather than dealing with the intense emotions created by our failure to find the intimacy we so desperately desire. Sometimes this preoccupation with food and eating can become an addiction, and we may find ourselves, our original needs still unmet, bound by powerful eating habits over which we seem to have no control.

Or we may starve ourselves, attempting to deny our hunger, redirecting our intense emotions into a relationship with food we can control. We try to make ourselves invulnerable to the painful, unfulfilled longings for intimacy by refusing to need anything at all, even food. We try to protect ourselves by becoming totally self-sufficient.

If our experience of intimacy was limited or distorted as we were growing up, we may know nothing of the inner security that true intimacy provides. We may find that our ability to give ourselves to another human being with the self-giving love that God intends is also impaired, and that even our relationship with God is tenuous or distorted.

Impediments to Intimacy

The intimacy for which we are created is disrupted when "something negatively influences or disrupts our relationship with another person."[5] This disruption ultimately affects our relationship with ourselves and with God. Intimacy can be breached when any (or a combination) of the following occurs:[6]

- *Rejection:* The person may have difficulty with relationships following rejection by an important person, such as a mother, father, grandparent, boyfriend or girlfriend, or close friend.
- *Death:* Intimacy is impeded when someone beloved to the person dies. When the person is not aware of the grieving process or is told or believes that grieving is not acceptable, the person does not grieve the loss of the relationship and move on.
- *Abuse:* Sexual (including incest, rape, date rape, or other sexually inappropriate behaviors), verbal, emotional, or physical abuse severely disrupt intimacy and have devastating and continuing effects on the person's relationship to self, others, and God.
- *Enmeshment:* Intimacy can be breached when a parent demands too close a relationship with a child. In turn, the child does not learn to set limits or to develop appropriate relationship skills with peers. (This will be discussed in chapter nine on boundaries.)
- *Abortion:* Some women with disordered eating have had one or more abortions. As a result, they may experience loneliness, shame, abandonment, and confusion, which keep them isolated and feeling guilty. These feelings may result from never having allowed themselves to grieve.
- *Adoption:* Any person who is adopted experiences a breach in intimacy. Adoptees may feel a "deep and persistent sense of abandonment and [may] show symptoms of unresolved grief. [They may] question [their] inherent value, wondering if something about [them] had been different, would [their] parents have chosen to raise [them]."[7] A mother who

gives up a child for adoption also experiences a breach in intimacy. She often wonders about the emotional impact of the adoption on her child and may frequently deny her own grief concerning the adoption.

If your eating is disordered, you have most likely been deeply hurt in one or more of these ways. Our need for intimacy is so strong that when it is denied, through the dysfunction of our families or some other traumatic event, we, in a desperate but misplaced attempt to insulate ourselves from the pain of the past, turn to food to help us avoid dealing with the intense pain of these emotional issues.

As you can see, our relationship with food, eating, and weight involves far more than whether or not we have the willpower to avoid a second helping or maintain a rigid diet. Hidden beneath the surface is our pain, our yearning, our ravenous desire to be loved, our longing to be cherished, to be protected, to belong, and to be valued and considered precious. As God's creations, we sense that we are made for relationship. We sense our need for an intimacy that will satisfy our need for security and significance, our need to be protected and cherished in relationship. We sense that we are made to be treated with dignity and respect. But instead, in a fallen world of broken relationships and dysfunctional family dynamics, we often receive deep emotional wounds that food will not heal.

Disordered eating does not satisfy our silent hunger. But according to the mercy of God, it will work to our good when we love him and are called according to his purpose. God takes this yearning, whether it is satisfied in our families or not, and sanctifies it. "After twenty years of listening to the yearnings of people's hearts, I am convinced that all human beings have an inborn desire for [intimacy with] God. Whether we are consciously religious or not, this desire is our deepest longing and our most precious treasure. It gives us meaning."[8] It is our silent hunger.

Our silent hunger does not go away. It may be repressed or suppressed, but it cannot be stifled. Ultimately our need for love, security, and significance must be satisfied. To do this we must, with

God's help, resurrect and confront whatever issues have caused us to turn to counterfeit substitutes for intimacy. As these issues are resolved we will be free to delight in the fullness of life God lovingly provides for us and to live a life of self-giving love that glorifies God forever. He restores us to freedom. We are healed.

Questions
(We suggest you keep a journal for addressing the questions at the end of each chapter.)

1. What is disordered eating?
2. Describe your disordered eating.
3. What are the causes of disordered eating?
4. List the possible causes of your disordered eating and how they have influenced your eating.
5. What is silent hunger and where does it come from?
6. What are the impediments to intimacy?
7. How have these impediments impacted your life?
8. What counterfeits have you turned to in attempting to satisfy your God-given need for intimacy?

Scripture to Read

1. 1 Samuel, chapters 18, 19, 20
2. Romans 7:7–25
*3. Romans 8:1–3

*We suggest that you commit this Scripture to memory.

Prayer

Dear God, I want to come to you with the things in my life that are both shameful and painful, but I am afraid. I feel both drawn to you and distant from you at the same time. I am hurting from keeping my thoughts, feelings, and behavior hidden and I need your help. I confess I have tried to fix things in my own strength, and I have failed miserably. I believe you want me to know you more intimately and I desire that as well, but it scares me because I am afraid that you will not love me when you see me as I really am. I confess I'm not sure where I stand with you right now. However, I ask you to take my hand and walk with me as I try to be honest, open, and intimate with you. Amen.

Invitation

Lord Jesus, I confess that I have been ambivalent and distant in my relationship with you. I desire to see you as my Comforter, Protector, Counselor, and Abba, Father. I have held back because of the rejection, pain, and hurts I experienced from my earthly family and people in general. My desire now is to have a personal relationship with you. I ask you to come into my heart as the Lord of my life and forgive me for all of my past failings, fears, and resentment. Wash me clean. I ask you to be my Savior as well, that I might rest in you and not try to earn my way but only receive what you have for me by your grace. Thank you that I don't have to be perfect in order to have this personal relationship with you. Thank you that I can come to you just as I am and that you receive me into your loving arms. Amen.

2

Resurrection Not Rigid Restraint

> When you repress or suppress those things which you
> don't want to live with, you don't really solve the prob-
> lem because you don't bury the problem dead—you bury
> it alive. It remains alive and active inside of you.
>
> John Powell
> *Why Am I Afraid to Love?*

Jesus said, "I am the resurrection and the life" (John 11:25).
God's gift to us is resurrection—restoration and recovery. Recovery from disordered eating is not only possible, it is what God intends. He brings life out of death, restores the broken, recovers the lost. Our faith in God's work frees us from the false belief that the only relief from disordered eating is lifelong deprivation, total abstinence, or adherence to fixed formulas that dictate what we can or cannot eat or how many calories we're allowed.

Many of us have tried diets, calorie counting, shots, or pills. We've been told to abstain from certain foods, such as refined sugar or white flour. The basic assumption of such approaches, which fail 95 percent of the time, is that the problem is either due to a simple lack of willpower or that certain foods are the cause of disordered eating. If only we change our behavior—abstaining or using another formula for weight loss—all of our problems with food will be solved.

Hoping to constrain, control, or at least manage our food, eating, and weight, we create entanglements that enslave us more. Even though we try to kill the hunger and bury the deeper emotional issues under our disordered eating, they are still alive and active inside us. The promise of the world is that if we will just restrain ourselves and restrict our intake, we will lose the weight and be set free. The pitfall in such promises is that they keep our focus on the formula for restraint, not on the God who has promised to restore us.

Restoration requires a life of faith—we believe we can be restored; a life of freedom—we risk stepping out of bondage to the past and our disordered eating; and a life of intimacy—we accept oneness with God and allow those appointed by God to participate in our restoration. But when we live a life based on fixed formulas of restraint, we plug ourselves into a rigid system, constantly fearful of failing. Eugene Peterson comments, "Any formula that prevents failure also prevents freedom."[1] When we allow God to work in us, speaking through our silent hunger, we begin to hear the promise of freedom.

"I have tried a well-known diet program countless times," says Rita. "For twenty years I would lose the weight, gain it back, lose it again. When I came to the Thin Within workshop I was rebellious. I didn't want to bring up the past; I just wanted someone to tell me what, when, and how much to eat. I struggled with knowing when I was hungry. In fact, it made me mad finally to realize that I would frequently eat when I wasn't hungry at all. When I began to pray about my relationship with food I realized that my silent hunger was my *loneliness*. I came from a family where there was alcohol abuse, physical abuse, and no intimacy. Food helped me survive. It was my comfort and my friend. After the workshop, I started thinking about going back to the diet pro-gram to quickly get the last twenty pounds off my body. 'When I'm thin I'll come back to this process,' I promised. But I realized this was a false promise. The truth was obvious: As I accepted the challenge of freedom and resolved the pain underneath, I would be free to enjoy a peaceful relationship with food and my body."

God gives us the freedom to observe and correct, to fail and succeed. Peterson continues, "He who has never failed some-where, that man cannot be great. Failure is the true test of great-ness."[2] Our greatness lies in our faith in God. He is always there to pick us up, and he continues walking with us until we have our ultimate freedom, when the underlying causes of our dis-ordered eating have been resolved. God's restoration is far more wonderful than the temporary resolution of our weight problem. It involves a complete recovery of our ability to eat and *live* as he intended. For this to happen we must allow God to move and to work in us, using the hunger we've tried in vain to satisfy. God wants to change our character for a higher purpose: to make us more like himself.

When God restores us, he respects and trusts the individual will and the freedom that he has given us. Our relationship with him is honored, because it is a life-giving process of discovery, not a process of success or failure based on our ability to follow a fixed formula. When God works his miracle of grace, he resurrects and empowers us to resolve the buried problem. But how will God resurrect us? How shall we be restored?

Resurrection (John 11:1–44)

"Now a man named Lazarus was sick. He was from Bethany, the village of Mary and her sister Martha" (v. 1). We don't know what he had, but whatever his illness, he was beyond the capac-ity to help himself. What we do know is that he was so sick that his sisters, deeply distressed over his condition, sent word to Jesus saying, "Lord, the one you love is sick" (v. 3). And we know that Lazarus was beloved by the Lord, a special friend, one with whom he had an intimate relationship.

"When he heard this, Jesus said, 'This sickness will not end in death. No, it is for God's glory, so that God's Son may be glorified through it.' Jesus loved Martha and her sister and Lazarus. Yet when he heard that Lazarus was sick, he stayed where he was for two more days" (vv. 4–6). Even though he loved Mary, Martha, and Lazarus, Jesus didn't drop everything and rush to heal Lazarus. He could have come immediately to the friends he loved, saving them much grief and anguish. He could have saved Lazarus from the ravages of a condition that put him in the tomb.

Like Lazarus, we are ravaged with the sickness of our disordered relationship with food, eating, and weight. Like Lazarus, we are not just an anonymous person in need but are intimate and special friends of the One who loves us. And like Lazarus we need divine help to be healed. But Jesus may not come immediately. He knows that as sick as we are this sickness need not end in death. Jesus knows that something great can come of it: "that God's Son might be glorified through it" (v. 4).

In spite of this, when he does finally arrive, we may, like Martha and Mary, think he is too late and blame him for his unconcern. Martha, hearing that Jesus was coming, went out to meet him. "Lord, if you had been here, my brother wouldn't have died" (v. 21). Maybe she clutched at his garments and implored, "Why didn't you come sooner? Why weren't you here? It's your fault that Lazarus is dead." We can almost hear Jesus' answer that she is worried and upset about too many things.

Then Mary, at home mourning, rose quickly and went out to meet Jesus. She fell at his feet. "Lord, if you had been here, my brother would not have died" (v. 32). Why did you let this happen? We thought you loved us. Mary and Martha, repeating the same phrase, expressed the heart's cry for protection. Why didn't you spare us this pain? "If you had been here, he wouldn't have died." Why must we suffer so? Jesus is deeply moved and grieved. We are told that he weeps.

"Then the Jews said, 'See how he loved him!'" (v. 36). Jesus' love for Lazarus and for us is not a distant or detached love, not a love meted out in abstract wishes for our own good from on high. Our Lord shares our suffering, weeping with us and for us in our pain, in our affliction, and in our grief. Our Lord enters into an intimate relationship with us, as he did with his beloved friend Lazarus, and that relationship does not spare him or us the anguish of loss or the reality of suffering. "We are healed of suffering only by experiencing it to the full."[3] Jesus knows this. Lazarus is proof.

> *Our Lord shares our suffering, weeping with us and for us in our pain, in our affliction, and in our grief.*

Scripture tells us simply, "The dead man came out" (v. 44a). Lazarus emerged from the dark tomb after lying dead for four days. He says nothing and does nothing. His face is covered, his hands and feet are bound. He can't see, he can't touch anyone, he can't move very well. "Take off the grave clothes and let him go," Jesus tells them (v. 44b). He doesn't address Lazarus. He doesn't tell Lazarus to take off his own grave clothes. He tells the friends and relatives and those who had been in mourning to take off the grave clothes. They are to restore Lazarus to his place in the community, to sight, touch, and wholeness.

Jesus called Lazarus from death to life, as he has done for each of us through his own death and resurrection. But now we may feel abandoned and entombed in the hopelessness of our disordered eating. We may feel some self-pity—that it is useless or that no one cares. We may stop seeking love, we may stop asking for intimacy, we may stop being emotionally available for close relationships. All that is left is our lifeless body, wrapped in the grave clothes[4] of our disordered eating, barricaded in our tomb, insulated and isolated from life. Like Lazarus, we may think we are beyond asking for help. But Jesus is there for us and does not hesitate: "Take away the stone," he said (v. 39).

We are alive in Christ; the saving work has been accomplished. But our grave clothes may still be in place, and if so, they can be removed only when we believe and have faith that we can be restored, when we risk stepping out of our tombs, and when we let our brothers and sisters participate in the unwrapping process. Jesus chooses to give certain people with whom we have relationships the privilege of participating in our restoration.

And that is what he does for us. He helps us to heal through restored intimacy by calling us into relationships where we must first rely on him and then on others to help unwrap the grave clothes. Thus our healing process becomes a marriage of the divine and the human. Divine power raised Lazarus and raises us from the dead, and human power unwrapped him and unwraps us. The spiritual and the physical reality combine to bring a complete healing.

We are not raised up out of our graves in perfection as Jesus was. Our resurrection is of a different order: We are raised with the same flawed bodies, disordered eating habits, and the same frailties from which we need help freeing ourselves. When Jesus brings us out of the tomb of our disorders, we may not initially be fit for company. We may not know how to relate very well, and we may have to learn some basic communication skills. We may have to develop new and appropriate coping techniques to replace the disordered behaviors of our past. All of this may be so threatening that we may want to back away from the unwrapping and keep those grave clothes bound around us. We may even want to flee back into the tomb and pull the stone over the entrance. How do we begin taking the steps toward intimacy?

The command of the Lord is that if we will prayerfully bring our needs before him, he will complete his work in us and preserve our dignity and humility in the process. "He who began a good work in you will carry it on to completion until the day of Christ" (Phil. 1:6).

Penetrating the Layers

"At one time we too were foolish, disobedient, deceived and enslaved by all kinds of passions and pleasures" (Titus 3:3). The apostle Paul speaks of those under the power of sin as deceived. The basis for the efficacy of deceit is its effect on the mind. "[Deceit] consists in presenting things to the mind in such a way that their true nature, causes, effects, or present conditions to the soul remain hidden."[5]

Deception

We are being deceived when we rely on our disordered eating to satisfy our silent hunger. Deception distorts our thinking, twisting our creative imagination to its purposes. The result is our inability to see the true nature of our condition. Deception precedes denial, and denial masks our disordered eating, allowing it to masquerade before us as a benign peculiarity or innocuous habit. In truth, disorders that flourish and become the focus of our lives keep us wrapped up and numbed, suppressing the unbearable tension of our unfulfilled inner needs. Deception keeps them in place, employing denial as its device.

Think about it. How many times have you told yourself, *I can eat whenever I want to—I'm not hurting anyone else. This is my body, and I can do what I want with it.* Or, *If I eat standing up, the food doesn't have as many calories.* Or, *I can have a second helping of pie and ice cream because I'll start my diet tomorrow.*

Years back when I (Judy) was working in a dental clinic, the patients would frequently bring us boxes of chocolates. I'd put as many as possible into a Kleenex, sneak into the darkroom, lock the door, and eat as if I were possessed. Then I'd come out and eat my salad for lunch and pretend to everybody that I was virtuous.

We get caught up in a vicious cycle, don't we? We are deceived; we deceive ourselves; we deceive others; we deny the reality of our behaviors and develop patterns of secrecy. Have you seen this cycle at work in your struggle with food, eating, and weight? Whenever there is dysfunction—whether in the past or in the present—deception, denial, and secrecy prevail.

Denial

Denial is a central controlling force in dysfunctional families, where those involved often live their lives pretending that reality is other than it really is. Our parents may have denied our experiences, our thoughts, and our feelings. We ourselves, having no accurate external reference, began to doubt and finally to deny the authenticity of our own experience.

"When I was in high school," says Claire, "I was extremely upset and very self-conscious because my weight got out of control. In my discouragement and shame, I told my mother how much I weighed. 'You shouldn't feel upset about that,' she told me. 'Just forget about it.' I knew what I felt, but my mother's words denied my experience."

Denial, like disordered eating, serves to block from our awareness feelings that appear unsafe to experience. Our denial may have originated when we were small and helpless as a coping mechanism, a defense to protect us against some awful truth that we were emotionally unable to face. It may have been too brutal, too terrifying, or too empty. And so to survive we began to shut down our feelings, eventually coming to the place where, in order to preserve that vulnerable self, we could not feel anything. We became incapable of trusting our experience and the signals our bodies sent us about that experience. Denying our experience, we denied our bodies. Denying our bodies, we denied life.

"My dad was an angry man," says Alexis, "and he would find fault with me as a way of venting his rage. I'd often feel trapped as he hovered over me shouting interminably about my behavior or some aspect of my appearance. It wasn't safe to show emotion—that only provoked him further—so I numbed my feelings and sort of left my body. I went dead. I'd hear his voice as if from a distance. It was my way of trying to avoid a frightening situation from which there seemed to be no escape."

Denial may have been how we learned to deal with reality in our dysfunctional families. It may have been our means of survival as we struggled to preserve our vulnerable selves from the ravages of extreme abuse, emotional cruelty, or neglect. But now it binds us, preventing the reemergence of healthy, appropriate responses to our pain and difficulty, both past and present. Unwrapping the grave clothes requires that we penetrate the layers of denial that conceal from us not only our past experiences but also our present behaviors. Deception and disordered eating hide from our minds the true nature of our condition, fomenting the denial that prevents us from experiencing and effectively dealing with the reality of our existence.

Unwrapping the Grave Clothes

Where denial darkens our path and compulsions hide and confine us, the light of God's love gently and compassionately penetrates the layers of our most ingrained defense mechanisms and coaxes us out of the tomb into the light. This light opens us to the possibility of intimacy, to the possibility of being transparent before God and yielding to his desire to help us see ourselves as we truly are—in need of tender mercy and in need of his glorious grace. "The gentleness of Jesus with sinners," writes Brennan Manning, "flowed from his ability to read their hearts. . . . [B]ehind people's most puzzling defense mechanisms . . . Jesus saw little children who hadn't been loved enough and who had ceased growing because someone had ceased believing in them."[6]

When we choose to allow the unwrapping of our grave clothes, we find a God who infinitely loves us and desires that we grow up into the fullness of the stature of Christ. But as we open the door to this light, we can expect disruption for a time. "I've been on a wild, emotional roller-coaster ride," says Karen, a woman who participated in a recent workshop. "I knew I had to go back to age six or seven and recall the sexual abuse. I had shoved the pain, sorrow, and shame as far down into my subconscious as possible. Now, examining my past, daily seeking God's grace, and letting go of the pain, I've discovered that, as heartbreaking and confusing as the process can be, as I empty out the old wounds, God fills me with more of himself."

Where once there was darkness and pain, we begin to see the light of life. This is the good news. Be assured that God does not ask us to unwrap the grave clothes all at once. He compassionately understands that denial has had a purpose in our lives, and he is gentle with us "for he knows how we are formed, he remembers that we are dust" (Ps. 103:14). He will not try us beyond what we are able to bear.

Once we are free to be unwrapped, to resurrect and resolve the issues beneath the surface, we can release our denial and defenses. As we do, God gives us the ability to value ourselves as he values us and to face, rather than hide from, the truth about ourselves. We are freed from the constriction of the shrouds that bind us, and we can expand into the breadth and depth of God's unfathomable love. His love gently coaxes us out into the light, wide-open spaces where we can enjoy the life he intends for us. "He reached down from on high and took hold of me; he drew me out of deep waters. . . . He brought me out into a spacious place" (Ps. 18:16, 19).

We may feel naked and vulnerable in this spacious place, and in a sense we are. The freedom that comes from allowing our grave clothes to be unwrapped is risky business. It is frightening, because intimacy threatens our comfort and challenges us to be more honest than perhaps we have been. It may seem easier to remain bound in our grave clothes and to accept counterfeits for intimacy. But those of us who are willing to risk intimacy and put ourselves in vulnerable positions with God and others must permit this process to unfold. We know we must die to come alive and that we must first suffer in order to be restored.

"Take courage! God often allows us to go through difficulties to purify our souls and to teach us to rely on him more. So offer him your problems unceasingly and ask him for the strength to overcome them. Talk to him often; forget him as seldom as possible. Praise him. When the difficulties are at their worst, go to him humbly and lovingly—as a child goes to a loving father—and ask for the help you need from his grace."[7]

Allowing our grave clothes to be unwrapped is an acknowledgment of our silent hunger, our desire for genuine intimacy. And genuine intimacy is often most available when least expected—at times of greatest unhappiness, profound loss, or uncontrollable tragedy. When confronted with such situations we have a choice: We can reach for the chocolate cake or ice cream, we can turn to friends and loved ones, or we can reach for our living God. The cake is temporarily predictable: It's there, and we know what it is going to taste like. Our friends are less predictable: They may not understand, they may reject us, or they may simply appease us. But God is another story.

The good news is we have a loving and all-powerful God, who is always predictable: "The Word became flesh and made his dwelling among us" (John 1:14). God is always there waiting with outstretched arms. He loves us. He will not misunderstand or reject us. He is consistent yesterday, today, and tomorrow. When we come to him with honesty and humility he establishes intimacy and relationship with us based on his love and mercy. He models intimacy, transparency, vulnerability, and communication with us in the person of his Son. God recognizes, above all, that we are incapable of intimacy apart from his love and our relationship with him, so he responds to us in our hour of greatest need.

Accepting Intimacy

Brennan Manning writes in *The Ragamuffin Gospel,* "Perhaps the simplest, though not the easiest place to start, is with myself. Carl Jung, the great psychiatrist, once reflected that we are all familiar with the words of Jesus, 'Whatever you do to the least of my brethren, that you do unto me.' Then Jung asks a probing question: 'What if you discovered that the least of the brethren of Jesus, the one who needs your love the most, the one you can help the most by loving, the one to whom your love will be most meaningful—what if you discovered that this least of the brethren of Jesus . . . *is you?*'"[8]

You. You are the one God invites out of your grave clothes and into an intimate relationship. We invite you to extend to yourself the intimacy and acceptance that God, in Christ, extends to you moment by moment.

Extending this intimacy to ourselves may be difficult because acceptance may not have been extended to us in our families of origin. We may have experienced ourselves as worthless because our families were critical, suspicious, ungrateful, controlling, inflexible, and shaming. But God offers us a relationship with a new family where we can experience ourselves as worthwhile. God's family is accepting, trusting, gentle, free, grateful, and confident[9] (see fig. 1).

Because of difficult and dysfunctional experiences as we grew up in our families, we may not be able to love and accept ourselves as God loves and accepts us. We may "lack the inner nurturing that could open [us] freely to others."[10]

When we come into an intimate relationship with God and others based on Christ's love for us, we begin to live beyond disordered eating. We are freed from our grave clothes. The profound intimacy provided to us by God in relationship with Christ stills our striving for things of this world and satisfies our silent hunger. "Then Jesus declared, 'I am the bread of life. He who comes to me will never go hungry, and he who believes in me will never be thirsty'" (John 6:35).

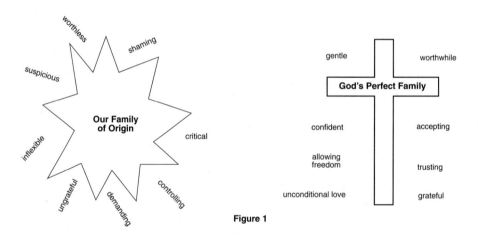

Figure 1

We can develop this intimacy and acceptance of ourselves only by seeing ourselves as God sees us. According to his Word we know that we are made in God's image;[11] chosen to be God's children;[12] bought at the infinitely valuable price of Christ's blood;[13] reconciled to God;[14] and heirs of God's kingdom.[15] We know that Jesus came so that we could have abundant life. Acceptance of ourselves involves appropriating that life by replacing our lack of self-acceptance and worth with God's gracious view of us. This enables us to accept our intrinsic, God-given value and to allow our grave clothes to be tenderly unwrapped. Do you believe that God's desire is to free you from the grave clothes that have kept you bound? Do you believe that he wants you to be a good steward of your body, which is the temple of the Holy Spirit? If you do, we invite you to begin now by rejecting the idea that your disordered eating will satisfy your silent hunger and accepting the truth that your security and significance come from experiencing an intimate relationship with God. Begin by accepting the gift of restoration. Live the life of faith, believing you can be restored. Step out of your tomb and live a free and intimate life. Experience oneness with God and allow those appointed by God to participate in the unwrapping of your grave clothes.

When we are restored to intimacy with God and receive his love, we become open to genuine intimacy with those around us. This allows us to experience a more complete sense of belonging, security, and significance. Intimacy with our living God allows us to unwrap our grave clothes, release our defenses, discard our counterfeit behavior, and come back to life. As we do, God gives us the ability and the strength to face, rather than hide from, the truth about ourselves. And when we truly believe that he loves and accepts us just as we are, we can then accept and love ourselves as we are. Renewed intimacy with God and ourselves quiets the insistent cry of our silent hunger and satisfies us in ways that nothing of this world or of our own doing can.

> *When we are restored to intimacy with God and receive his love, we become open to genuine intimacy with those around us.*

God meets our deepest desire for intimacy in *relationship*. We find a deep sense of security and significance based on God's image of us, knowing we are accepted by God *as we are*. The more fully we embrace this truth and accept ourselves, with all our flaws and frailties, the more completely our silent hunger will be satisfied and the greater will be our sense of peace.

In the chapters that follow we will look at the basic principles that will enable you to begin to hear the voice of your silent hunger. When God restores you, he helps you resolve painful past experiences and replace old unworkable beliefs with right thinking. You will find that your mind and heart will be renewed by the power of the Holy Spirit. Disordered eating will be replaced with the ability to eat as God intended you to eat. Your silent hunger will be satisfied as you receive the truth of God's unconditional love for you.

"Then you will know the truth, and the truth will set you free" (John 8:32). Removing our grave clothes brings us to truth. When we know the truth, we are freed from our attempts to fill our need for intimacy with food rather than with our living God. We are freed from our distorted view of God and ourselves, and we are freed for the true intimacy that will allow us to receive and give genuine life-giving love. To begin, you must be willing to allow your grave clothes to be removed, to give voice to your silent hunger, and to listen to yourself, body, mind, and soul in the presence of God.

Are you ready and willing to risk stepping into the light of freedom? Take courage. We know it is difficult to have the grave clothes unwrapped, layer by layer, painful fold by painful fold. But remember: God is in control of this process, and he will comfort and sustain you. His Word and his Spirit will be your constant companions.

Unwrapping our grave clothes is risky and requires courage, but it is necessary and rewarding. For we "who, with unveiled faces all reflect the Lord's glory, are being transformed into his likeness with ever increasing glory, which comes from the Lord, who is the Spirit" (2 Cor. 3:18). This is our high calling. This is our hope.

Please read "Reconciling with Your Body" and follow instructions for "The Body Awareness Exercise" in the additional resources section.

Questions

1. What is required in order to be "restored"?
2. What was most meaningful to you about the story of Lazarus being raised from the dead?
3. What is meant by "grave clothes"?
4. List anything in your life that might be considered grave clothes.
5. Who would you be willing to have help you remove your grave clothes?
6. With whom can you share your innermost feelings and thoughts? Do you feel comfortable doing this? If not, why not?
7. How does deception contribute to your disordered eating?
8. How does denial contribute to your disordered eating?
9. What happens when we choose to allow our grave clothes to be removed?
10. In your journal describe your earthly family of origin.
11. In your journal describe your perfect family of God.
12. How does God see you?
13. How do you see yourself?
14. What can we look forward to when God restores us?

Scripture to Read

1. Genesis 1:27
2. Psalm 103
3. John 1:12, 6:35, 8:32, and 11:1–44
4. Romans 8:29
*5. 1 Corinthians 6:19–20
6. Ephesians 1:4
7. 1 Peter 1:20 and 2:9
8. 1 John 3:1

*We suggest that you commit this Scripture to memory.

Prayer

Dear God, thank you that you are a sovereign God. You know all things. You know the behaviors in my life that are not pleasing to you or to me. I realize that some of these behaviors stem from issues in my life that I have tried desperately to bury, and I recognize that nothing is hidden from your eyes. The pain of trying to hide these things has become too much for me to bear, and I humbly ask you to prepare me to see the truth behind my behavior, so I can be set free. I ask this in Jesus' name. Amen.

Part **2**

===================

Free
to Change

3

Grace Not Legalism

God is infinitely patient. He will not push Himself into our lives. He knows the greatest thing He has given us is our freedom, for therein lies our power to love. He respects our freedom. If we want habitually, even excessively, to operate at the level of our own reason, He will respectfully keep silent. We can fill ourselves with our own thoughts, ideas, images and feelings. He will not interfere. But if we invite Him with attention, opening the inner space with silence, He will begin to speak to our souls, not in words or concepts, but in the mysterious way that love expresses itself—by presence.

M. Basil Pennington
Centered Living

Our freedom is expressed most fully in the glory of grace—the intimate, spontaneous, and absolute loving-kindness of God working in us to make us whole. "Grace is the active expression of God's love. Grace empowers us to choose rightly in what seem to be the most choiceless of situations, but it does not, and will not, determine that choice."[1] Grace influences our innermost being, bringing our character into agreement with the very character of God. This intimate acquaintance of our will with God's will, our spirit with God's Spirit, is a miracle, the miracle of God's presence perfecting our personal transformation. Grace is freedom that conforms us from within; legalism is bondage that constrains us from without.

Grace is freedom that conforms us from within; legalism is bondage that constrains us from without.

Legalism says that we must shape up by adhering to fixed formulas or a rigid set of laws or codes. This is a deception, however, because no external constraint (legalism) can satisfy our need for love and intimacy, nor can it create a pure heart.

From the beginning of salvation history, we have witnessed the interplay of law and grace. We saw God establishing a covenant with his chosen people, Israel, setting before them the laws that prescribed the form and content of behavior befitting a relationship with the Holy of Holies—laws and observances intended to initiate and establish a relationship between God and his people (see Exodus 19:5; 20:20; 21:1; 24:3). Knowing nothing of how to live in relationship with this God, Israel needed the law to teach them what was expected and to constrain their behaviors so that their lives were consistently brought back, by observance of the law, to a right relationship with God (see Leviticus 18:4–5).

But rather than successfully constraining behavior, the law demonstrated the impossibility of ever conforming perfectly to God's standards. The law "offers a limited, defined, explicit morality which localizes the sin in a particular action or particular unclean thing. It claims to give man a salvation which he can win for himself by strict observance, and in reality it plunges him into irremediable distress. . . . Progressive revelation, beginning with the prophets and culminating in Jesus, paints a different picture: [it] places guilt in the heart of man and not in things, in the intention, in being, not in doing. [This] proclaims the unlimited character of God's requirements, and the subsequent impossibility for man to wipe out his guilt by the perfection of his moral conduct."[2]

Throughout Scripture and throughout our lives, particularly as we wrestle with disordered eating, we witness the failure of our attempting to come into right relationship with God through our own efforts. We are powerless to achieve genuine goodness by flawless behavior, because our hearts are not pure. Where does this leave us? Paul's discussion on the law in Romans reveals that the purpose of the law was never to make us righteous but to reveal the depth of our own sin and to demonstrate our need of a Savior (see Romans 3:19ff and Galatians 3:1–20). "The answer, then, comes from God, not from man, in the forgiveness He grants to those who confess their inevitable guilt instead of justifying themselves."[3]

Let's return to Hannah for a moment to see how the dynamics of self-justification, forgiveness, and grace were revealed in her life. "In my marriage I justified rejecting love by saying, 'My father never loved me, I assume I'm not going to be loved,' so I'm no longer going to invest any of myself in this marriage.' But more significant was my attitude that my husband was blowing it anyway by his affairs, so he didn't deserve any effort from me. I had no sense of my participation in our deteriorating relationship. I was blaming the breach between us on his adultery, when in fact part of the responsibility was mine. Part of the distance between us came from my unspoken message, 'I know you will never love me enough or in the right way.' My justification kept me locked into refusing to admit my own guilt. Until I was willing to acknowledge it, I had no capacity to be reconciled to him. When I finally did confess my guilt to him, it was too late, as he no longer wanted the marriage to be restored. But I received reconciliation anyway, because in my brokenness God began to work in me and my capacity to receive love. And God has been working within me ever since. I had to confess that my backing out of intimacy was my choice and had nothing to do with whether or not the other person was being loving. Recognizing and confessing that particular dynamic with my husband made it possible for me to receive God's grace."

"Grace is the dynamic outpouring of God's loving nature that flows into and through creation in an endless self-offering of healing, love, illumination, and reconciliation," writes Gerald May.[4] And this dynamic outpouring was made flesh in Jesus Christ. Christ became the new offering—the means of atonement and reconciliation—for our sin and guilt. The law opened the way for God's grace. "For those who are in Christ Jesus. . . the law of the Spirit of life set [us] free from the law of sin and death. For what the law was powerless to do in that it was weakened by the sinful nature, God did by sending his own Son in the likeness of sinful man to be a sin offering" (Rom. 8:1–3).

So, we are no longer under the law, but we have received the gift of grace so that "the righteous requirements of the law might be fully met in us" (Rom. 8:4). When we receive this grace, through faith, a paradoxical shift occurs in our lives. Whereas we formerly were unable to live righteously by the law's constraints, we now begin to be conformed from within to the intent of the law, which is God's will for us. God, in his grace, not only offers forgiveness, but gives us the power, through faith in the indwelling Christ, to become sons and daughters—bearers of his character and will. God strengthens you "with power through his Spirit in your inner being, so that Christ may dwell in your hearts through faith . . . [and] that you, being rooted and established in love may have power . . . to know this love that surpasses knowledge" (Eph. 3:16–19).

It is this love, this outpouring of God's grace, that works the transformation of our innermost being so that we delight in pleasing him—indeed, live to please him. When we love Christ and our desire is to please him in everything, we are released from clinging to rules, regulations, and performance. We experience a profound freedom and at the same time are given the power to live out that freedom, for Christ sent the Holy Spirit to enable us to live, not by the letter of the law, but by its spirit, and its spirit is love. "Love is the fulfillment of the law" (Rom. 13:10), the law embodied in one word. To be under grace, then, is not a matter of being constrained by legalism but of being embraced by God's very essence, which is love, and its active expression, which is grace.

The question we must ask ourselves as we encounter grace in our lives is, Shall we risk living by it? Shall we place our faith in the free, spontaneous, and absolute loving-kindness of God working in us to make us whole, or shall we continue to live by legalistic systems?

"I feel safe and secure when I'm told what to eat and don't have to think about it," says Rebecca. "I both love and hate counting calories and weighing and measuring my food. On the one hand, I feel like I'm really doing something righteous, but on the other hand it gets so tedious, and I feel so guilty when I fail that I tend to give up in despair."

In the case of those of us who struggle with disordered eating, the standard of legalism might be to be "thin," to achieve a certain weight at all costs, or the belief that when we "lose" weight, life will be perfect and we will be free from all our problems. When we adopt external methods to constrain our behavior, we are buying the lie that victory can be won with our self-will. While "losing weight" may result in an immediate increase in our sense of self-worth and value, it is temporary and does not change the deep-rooted feeling that we are irredeemably flawed nor does it satisfy our silent hunger for intimacy with God.

If we are not secure in our own godly worth, we may try to conform externally by scanning the environment for cues and then adjusting our behavior accordingly. For instance, we may be obsessive about being known as a noneater, or as a "good" person. "Sometimes when I'm with a group of people, I won't eat because I don't want to look like a hungry person," says Lisa. "Then, of course, when I go home I eat far more than I really want, because, in an effort to look good, I publicly denied myself food when I was actually hungry. I let the external pressures overrule my body's internal message."

We even may take these attempts at external regulation a dangerous step further. Our compulsive behaviors themselves, exhibited in our disordered relationships with food, eating, and weight, can be described as an external regulation by a "self-defined system of control, safety, and security."[5] In short, legalism. Do you see how we ourselves can set up the most legalistic system of all in our self-protective relationship with food? By focusing on externals—our diets, our weight, our eating or not eating—we avoid confronting the real issues in our lives: our fears, unresolved grief, emotions, relationships, rebellion, and insecurities. By imposing self-discipline and losing some weight, we obtain a self-awarded victory that may temporarily provide us with a false sense of superiority or significance. In the process, however, we become self-satisfied and further repress our awareness of the real issues beneath our low self-esteem or discontentedness. In this condition, we refuse to allow the grave clothes to be unwrapped and therefore fail to acknowledge that it is in our *being* (the intentions of own hearts), not in our *doing* (our eating) that our true guilt lies.

Just as obedience to the law, an external mechanism for establishing righteousness, did not remove our guilt, our focus on an external, self-regulated coping mechanism does not remove our deepest problems. In our struggle with food, eating, and weight, there is no law, no diet, no deprivation we can summon that will subdue our compulsive indulgence. Not only can we not control or restore equilibrium to our lives by imposing external regulations, but also because we focus only on the symptoms, the *doing* only, we actually inflame our eating behaviors further. "Since you died with Christ to the basic principles of this world, why, as though you still belonged to it, do you submit to its rules: 'Do not handle! Do not taste! Do not touch!' These are all destined to perish with use, because they are based on human commands and teachings. Such regulations indeed have an appearance of wisdom, with their self-imposed worship, their false humility and their harsh treatment of the body, but they are of no value against the indulgence of the flesh" (Col. 2:20–23). We indulge the flesh (the self estranged from God) when we eat to mask the emotions with which we feel unable or unwilling to deal. You have experienced this yourself if you struggle with excessive dieting, compulsive overeating, or bulimia: you almost always binge after dieting or "losing" weight. For every rigid diet, there is an opposite kick-back binge. Or a binge may follow a day-long abstinence when your appetite rears its head and demands to be appeased.

Our silent hunger lies deep within: Rules don't affect it, diets don't change it, and legalism can't cure it. Until our focus shifts from *doing* (diets, food, eating, and weight) to *being* (the intentions of our hearts), we will fail to admit the gravity of our guilt. When we attempt to rely on our disordered eating to cover our deepest fears, hurts, and insecurities, we miss the opportunity to experience the miracle of intimacy from God's grace that can come only when we approach him as our Abba, Father, and depend on him and him alone. "Those whom God welcomes with open arms are not the virtuous, but the despised, not those who deny their guilt, but those who confess it. Repentance is the door to grace."[6]

"After I took the Thin Within workshop, I gave my life to the Lord and began couples counseling with my husband," says Alexis. "I had struggled with compulsive eating for years, but I had never looked further than the next diet trying to find a solution to my problem. After several sessions and with much fear and hesitation I was able to confess to my husband about an affair I'd had twelve years before. After his initial shock and indignation, he was able to forgive me. I was so relieved, and I felt released from the burden of guilt and shame I had carried for years. Our relationship is gradually moving to a deeper level of intimacy, and I am finding that more and more I am eating in response to my physiological hunger rather than in response to the tension produced by the guilt I lived with for so many years."

Grace is "receiving a gift with open hands"; legalism is "keeping rules with clenched fists."[7] Grace evokes in us a desire to *conform;* legalism provokes our desire to *perform.* Grace allows us to *be;* legalism compels us to *do.* Grace involves response-ability; legalism imposes solutions. Grace redirects our focus away from *perfection* to *correction.* When we strive for perfection, we attempt to master and control life by trying to measure up to some external, idealized standard. Striving for perfection, we are living the lie that we can make ourselves more acceptable to ourselves, to others, and to God if we just follow the letter of the law. Under grace we are free to turn to God as we really are, free to learn from our mistakes, free to change and grow, and free to allow him to help us become all he intends us to be. Under legalism our response is "have to"; under grace it is "want to." Under grace we respond out of love, out of our desire to please the one who first loved us. Our inclination springs from a heart yearning to respond to our loving God.

Thin Within Principles

We have seen that our reliance on legalistic practices such as diets, calorie counting, or other external weight-control measures fails to resolve our disordered eating because it fails to address the real issues. In fact, it only makes things worse. In using a grace-oriented approach to our bodies and our struggles with food, we are released from our tenacious tendency to wrap ourselves up in rules, regulations, and performance. We can then experience the outpouring of God's grace and are given the freedom and the power to develop a new relationship with food, eating, and our weight. Through grace we can begin to honor the natural response to our body's hunger signals and our ability to be satisfied with an appropriate amount of food. By grace we relinquish our reliance on legalistic controls that circumvent our bodies' messages, and we cultivate a moment-by-moment attentiveness to the Holy Spirit within us as we are conformed and transformed to a new identity in Christ.

What does this mean? It means that you are about to abandon legalism and learn an entirely new way of relating to food, eating, and your body. It means that you can develop the ability to eat what, when, and how much God directs you to eat. During this process you will rediscover the delights of good food and experience the joy of being the size God designed you to be. This new relationship is characterized by honor for the temple of the Holy Spirit—your body. In honoring your body you are guided by principles that support the delight you have in good food and the pleasure you enjoy in partaking of God's gifts. "Therefore glorify God in your body" (1 Cor. 6:20 KJV).

Imagine that you have a beloved friend who knows you better than you know yourself and that this friend desires that you have only the best. Now, imagine this friend saying, "I want you to live life to the full, and that includes eating the foods you enjoy and being the size God designed you to be. Here's the way to do it." The following principles for weight mastery will help set you free.

1. **Eat only when my body is hungry.** This is the essential principle for weight mastery. If you're not sure you are hungry or you are only a little bit hungry, then wait until your body signals true hunger. "But," you say, "how do I know when I'm truly hungry? I'm always hungry, and I always eat when I feel hungry. If I don't, I become ravenous, I faint, or I get a headache." Don't worry. We understand your frustration and will address your concerns later on in the book. Remember for the moment that physiological hunger is a God-given response to your body's need for food. You will find that when you listen attentively to your body's messages, your response will be clear. When you honor your body's signals and treat your body as an honored partner, you can release excess weight. When you "lose" weight, you "find" it again. How many times have you found those pounds you had lost? When you *release* weight, you say goodbye and you let it go forever.

2. **Reduce the number of distractions in order to eat in a calm environment.** Give your body the pleasure of a peaceful and serene environment in which to savor food. When you do this you also give yourself the opportunity to listen to your body's messages. You will begin to know what foods you really enjoy eating, experience more pleasure eating these foods, and you will know when it's time to stop. Turn off the television, put away the book, clear the newspaper off the table. You are in good company. Enjoy the relationship!

3. **Eat only when I'm sitting.** When you sit down at the table with your meal, you will be much more likely to engage in present-time eating, fully cognizant of what, when, and how much you eat, than if you eat on the run or graze through the kitchen cupboards. Eat in present time, not in the whirl of emotional upheaval generated by past events. When you don't fully enjoy the food in the present, you frequently come back for seconds. Remember also that when you eat on the run or while

standing at the kitchen counter, you are more likely to discount the fact that you have eaten. Your mind may erase the memory of the meal, but your body won't.

4. **Eat only when my body and mind are relaxed.** Pause before you plunge into your meal. Give thanks for what God has provided, and then prepare yourself to enjoy fully the eating experience. Allow all of your senses to come into play. Smell the food; let your eyes take in the colors and the arrangement on your plate. The point is you will enjoy the eating experience much more if you have allowed all your senses to savor the delight of the food. It will taste much better and satisfy you more than you could have imagined.

5. **Eat and drink only the food and beverages that I enjoy.** No more "Do not handle! Do not taste! Do not touch!" You are free to choose to eat *anything* you enjoy eating—as long as you eat only when you are hungry and stop *before* you are full (this will be discussed in more detail later in the chapter). Your body will tell you exactly what it requires. You're in an honoring partnership now, and when you listen to your body, you can trust it to respond appropriately.

But, you may say, what if my body wants only those forbidden foods that make me fat? And what about cholesterol? Barring medical constraints, you are free to choose any foods you enjoy eating. You are abandoning legalistic structures. You are living out of the profound freedom of the Spirit, which will guide your choices and actions if you listen attentively. Your body will *not* always want chocolate cream pie or french fries. Sooner or later you will notice as this process unfolds that your body will delight more in the foods that it requires for health and vigor.

6. **Pay attention only to my food while eating.** Easy enough when you're eating alone, but what about when you are with a friend or socializing? You will begin to establish a new rhythm—like a dance—when eating and socializing. First, focus on your meal, then put your fork down and focus on your friend and conversation. You will enjoy the entire experience of eating and relating more when you allow yourself to give your full attention first to one and then the other. Both your body and your relationships will benefit from the intimacy engendered in the

exchange. This may require some creativity, particularly with small children, but it is possible. (There is further information in the Medical Issues and Family Eating Patterns in the Additional Resources section at the end of the book.)

7. **Eat slowly, savoring each and every bite.** This is an opportunity for "eating meditation." We so often rush through the day not noticing the small (or large) delights in the people or things around us. When you slow down and focus your full attention in the present moment, you are saying to God and to your body, *I am living in the present, joyfully receiving the good gifts of creation and giving thanks for my ability to enjoy what I have received.* We honor God when we honor ourselves as the creation he has made.

8. **Stop before my body is full.** "There is a time for everything, and a season for every activity under heaven" (Eccles. 3:1). Just as we learned not to eat until we were truly hungry, so we honor our bodies by stopping when we have had just enough to be satisfied. This may sound difficult, and it is challenging, but it is possible. (It simply requires a bit of practice.) By doing this you give your body a rest, a chance to complete its natural digestive cycle before eating again. If you honor your body by waiting for it to signal true hunger, you will more easily be able to recognize when you are at that "comfortable" point when it's time to stop eating.

These principles apply to all the food you eat and all the beverages you drink, *except* water. Coffee, tea, alcohol, and diet sodas are included, because everything, except water, affects your body's ability to register accurately its physiological hunger.

At this point you may be thinking, *This is just another set of rules! I thought legalistic systems were out.* The principles are not fixed formulas or rigid rules. They are guidelines that involve choices. To be under grace is freedom—we have the privilege of seeing God's design for ordered eating and then choosing. God honors us with the freedom to fail and succeed as we risk living a life of faith. As we begin to practice the principles, we will see that God is calling us to surrender to a growing up, a maturing process. This is a challenge that calls us to have the courage to step out of our grave clothes of legalism and allow God to conform us from within.

The principles preserve our freedom because they respect the truth of how God made our bodies. They reflect our natural, God-given ability to determine our hunger and to choose to satisfy it appropriately. Do you know any people who exhibit these principles in their behavior? Think of people you know who appear to maintain their natural size with ease. What do these people do when they are hungry? Maybe they choose to eat pizza at lunch time, but they probably don't eat a whole one. Or perhaps they eat only half of a luscious dessert, leaving the rest for later (a remarkable feat). These principles are consistently observed by people who are not obsessed with or bound by any external constraints in regard to food and eating. The principles are an invitation to engage in eating behavior that, without constraining us, will conform us from within because they permit us to treat our bodies with the same high regard that God has for us.

> *To be under grace is freedom—we have the privilege of seeing God's design for ordered eating and then choosing.*

Children, too, are excellent role models of this type of eating behavior. They naturally practice these principles, being very clear about what they want to eat and eating only as much as they want. These children are *you* before your eating habits were influenced or determined by layers and layers of old patterns, beliefs, and inappropriate responses to life's stresses. The principles are nothing you don't know already; you have simply forgotten or wrapped them in the grave clothes of past conditioning.

Remember, this is not a diet. We are shifting the focus from legalism to grace and inviting you to be aware of *when* you eat and *how much*. The principles for weight mastery allow you the freedom to eat the foods you really enjoy *and* to be the size that God designed you to be. You will find that you can eat *what* you want *and* release weight at the same time when you allow these principles to guide you.

While you are learning to make new choices and establish new habits, it is a good idea to post these principles in an obvious location, such as on the refrigerator door! They will help you at critical times.

The Hunger Scale

Now that you know the eight principles for weight mastery, the next step is to begin to practice listening to your body and be led by the Spirit to distinguish between hunger and appetite. As the grave clothes are peeled away, you will more easily be able to recognize the difference between the two. Hunger is a sensation in the body caused by the need for food. Appetite is a habitual desire for some gratification, either of the body or the mind, that has nothing to do with true physiological hunger. Our hunger can be satisfied; our appetite is insatiable. Hunger looks to food to satisfy an appropriate *physical* need; appetite looks to food to satisfy *emotional* needs.

In Thin Within we use the Bodometer Process to determine our true hunger. This is a tool for turning our attention inward and listening to the signals our bodies are giving us in order to determine whether food (or something else) is needed. Your God-given physiological hunger is a clear message that you will be able to hear as you persevere in listening for it.

The following simple exercise introduces you to the Bodometer Process. First read through the exercise, then close your eyes and begin:

Sit in a comfortable position with your eyes closed. Focus your attention on the area of your mouth and teeth. Are there any sensations there that you would call hunger, time to eat, just comfortable, or stuffed? Focus your attention on your throat. What sensations do you experience in your throat? With what do you associate these sensations? Focus your attention on your stomach. What sensations do you experience in your stomach? With what do you associate these sensations? Focus your attention on your abdomen, the area just below your stomach. What sensations do you experience in your abdomen? With what do you associate those sensations? Place your hands on your stomach and abdomen. On a scale of "0" to "10," "0" being "empty," "5" "comfortable," and "10" "stuffed," at what level of hunger is your body right now in present time?

As you reflect on this exercise you will begin to recognize that true hunger sensations come only from your stomach, not from your mouth, your throat, or anywhere else. Sensations in your mouth and throat are real, but they have nothing to do with hunger. Even a growling stomach does not necessarily mean that you are hungry. It may be in the process of digesting food from your last meal, or it may just be reacting to stress or tension. This is a time to let your stomach complete its cycle and then return to rest before you eat again. Some people say that if their stomachs growl once, they think they are hungry. We often mistakenly think that any sensation between our chin and our knees is a call for food.

Your "0" is the only accurate indicator of true physiological hunger. You may not have a clue as to what your hunger signals are, however. This is not uncommon. Many workshop participants report never having experienced true hunger. Many ask, "How can I be sure I am at a '0'?" It may take some time and practice, but you will be able to recognize your "0," that clear signal of physiological hunger, if you are willing to wait. If you are not sure you are there, you can trust that you are not. In other words, when in doubt, don't eat! Your body will send a clear message that it's time to eat when you are at a "0." Sometimes hunger can be like a snooze alarm: it fades in and out until finally the signal is constant and clear. That's your "0." It won't be a *maybe* or *sort of,* it will be a definite *yes!*

The hunger scale on the following page is a visual representation of your body's physiological hunger level. The desired goal is to eat between a "0" and a "5."

What does recognizing your hunger number have to do with weight mastery? The hunger scale is a graphic representation to assist you in releasing weight. If you eat from "0" to "5" on the hunger scale, you will release weight until you are down to your natural, God-given size, and you will maintain that size. If you

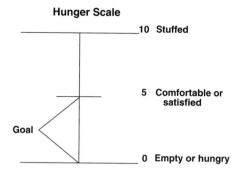

Figure 2

eat starting at "3" and continue eating to a "7" on the hunger scale, you will remain overweight. And if you eat from a "5" up to "10" on the hunger scale, you will gain weight.

As you use the Bodometer Process daily you will become better at knowing where you are on your internal hunger scale. It will become a valuable tool in your weight mastery process. It will become a way of life.

How much food does it take to bring us to a comfortable "5" or less? Make a fist. This is the approximate size of your stomach when it is empty. Yes, we know this is a real shock. You can see how little food you actually need to fill this space. In addition to

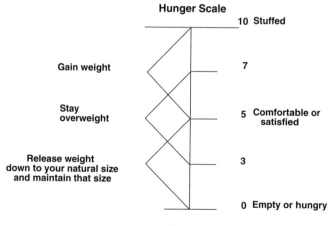

Figure 3

the hunger scale, you can use your fist as a reminder of how much to eat. As one workshop participant said, "It's always right in front of my face, wrapped around my fork!"

Using the language of "0" or empty, rather than saying you are "starving" or "famished," takes the fear out of allowing yourself not to eat. Remember, you won't starve. Think of Jesus in the wilderness. After forty days and forty nights he said, "I'm hungry." We're not suggesting that you go without food for forty days, but we are saying that you can safely wait until you are certain you are hungry before you eat, which might mean skipping a meal once in a while. As we change our language, we can change our responses and establish new, healthy ways of responding to our bodies' messages.

The beauty of the hunger scale is that it helps us differentiate between hunger and appetite. We can assess our hunger by checking in with our body (Bodometer Process) to see where we are from "0" to "10" on our internal hunger scale. If we are at a "0," we can eat—until we reach a comfortable "5." On the other hand, if we're experiencing appetite, food isn't and never will be the answer, and we *can* choose not to eat. Once we acknowledge the difference between true hunger and appetite, we are free to make loving choices that will address our specific needs.

The hunger scale helps us to listen and respond appropriately to our bodies' natural cycle of hunger and satiation. As we continue this process and experience God's healing of our silent hunger, we will release weight and be transformed from the inside out to be the size and the spiritual temple God intended us to be.

We no longer rely on our bathroom scales to tell us when we've eaten too much and gained weight (more about scales in chapter four). We no longer count calories to regulate our daily intake. We no longer rely on legalism that constrains us from without. We now rely on God's grace—the freedom that conforms us from within. This takes courage!

What is it that attracts us to legalism? Recall the story of the Israelites coming out of Egypt. They were in the wilderness, having been set free from the bondage of slavery, and they had the assurance of God's presence in their midst. What did they do? They started grumbling, and some of them even wanted to return to Egypt. "If only we had died by the Lord's hand in Egypt! There we sat around pots of meat and ate all the food we wanted, but you have brought us out into this desert to starve this entire assembly to death" (Exod. 16:3). Maybe we are like the Israelites. Our newly acquired freedom may be unsettling, even frightening. At first we may not trust it. We may be tempted to go back to the bondage, sitting around the "pots of meat"—the meal plans—to have something external dictating when, what, and how much we should eat. Only by means of God's freedom will we begin to learn the precious lessons of trust and surrender that will ultimately lead to the maturity of body, mind, and soul he desires for us. We must begin to live by faith and not by the law. "It is for freedom that Christ has set us free. Stand firm, then, and do not let yourselves be burdened again by a yoke of slavery" (Gal. 5:1).

Questions

1. What is God's grace?
2. How does God's grace work in our lives?
3. What is legalism? How does it affect our lives?
4. What was the purpose of God's law?
5. In your journal write down the legalistic methods you have tried in attempting to resolve your weight and eating problems.
6. List the Thin Within principles for weight mastery. How do you plan to implement each of these principles in your life?
7. How do the principles differ from legalism (diets, calorie counting, etc.)?
8. What is the Bodometer Process?
9. What is the hunger scale and how can it serve you?
10. What attracts us to legalism?
11. Record your hunger number from the time you awaken in the morning until going to sleep at night, noting particularly what your number is just before and after you eat. In the sample graph on the following page, the person ate from "0" to "5" at breakfast (8 A.M.), "2" to "8" at lunch (1 P.M.), and "1" to "6" at dinner (7 P.M.). (Ideally you would start at "0" and stop at "5.") It will help you

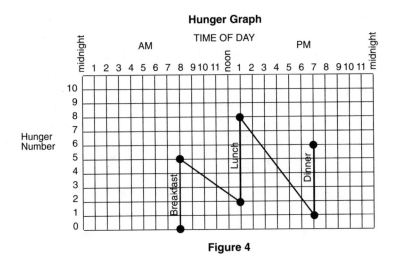

Figure 4

to make a copy of this graph and use it until "0" to "5" eating becomes second nature.

Scripture to Read

1. Psalm 140
*2. Romans 3:10–20, 4:13–17, and 5:20–21
3. Galatians 3:1–20
4. Colossians 2:20–23

*We suggest that you commit this Scripture to memory.

Prayer

Dear God, thank you for my body, which is lovingly and wonderfully made by you. I marvel that it still supports me even after all the abuse I have heaped on it. I confess that I still dislike parts of my body. I regard them as less than acceptable. I have trouble separating their strengths and usefulness from the excess weight I have put on as a result of my compulsive eating. By your grace, help me to put aside the critical thoughts with which I have been judging my body. Grant me acceptance and appreciation for the marvelous creation you have made me to be. In your name I ask that you heal my body, mind, and soul. Amen.

4

=====================================

Conscious
Eating Not
Compulsive
Eating

If man is constantly exiled from his own home, locked out of his spiritual solitude, he ceases to be a true man. He is not even a healthy animal. He becomes a kind of automaton, living without joy because he has lost all spontaneity. He is no longer moved from within, but only from outside himself. He no longer makes decisions for himself, he lets them be made for him. He no longer acts upon the outside world, but lets it act upon him. He is propelled through life by a series of collisions with outside forces. His is no longer the life of a human being, but the existence of a sentient billiard ball, a being without purpose and without any deeply valid response to reality.

Thomas Merton
The Silent Life

It takes courage to receive freedom. It takes courage to change. We may prefer to exist in the security of our grave clothes—our diets, our disordered eating, our buried, but not dead, past. How do we make the transition from bondage to freedom, from fixed formulas to using the Thin Within principles and living in the freedom and acceptance God intends for us?

When Scripture describes freedom, it describes a God who sets the captives free—he delivers his people from bondage. The word *deliver* "denotes not a removal from, but a rescue from the power of."[1] When we are rescued from the power of all that protected, or seemed to protect us before now, we can lay bare our souls and surrender to the presence of God. When we do, we begin to attend to ourselves and God in the present moment. Having our attention, God continues his gentle but persistent work, restoring us to freedom and inviting us to respond in a whole and healthy way to the reality of our lives.

Being free does not remove us from the world of images, diets, or temptations to disordered eating. Instead, in our freedom God rescues us from the power of our past and from the power our disordered eating seems to hold over our lives. He rescues us from the things that prevent us from living by faith and from those things that stand in the way of our applying the principles.

Fat Machinery

The things that will stand in the way of applying the principles and using the hunger scale are behaviors we call "fat machinery." Fat machinery is unconscious, automatic, or inappropriate eating that is activated by external or internal stimuli. What this means is that much of our eating is done for the wrong reasons—social pressure, anxiety, frustration, and a variety of emotional stimuli that have nothing to do with our body's need for nourishment. When we are wrapped up in our grave clothes, our eating is activated by these stimuli and we move through life like robots or automatons, reaching for food unconsciously when something or someone activates our "eat" button.

"When I heard the principles in the workshop," says Lisa, "I thought, *It makes no sense that I should wait for my '0' before eating. I know how to tell when I'm hungry. Have I had my four square meals today? No? Then I'm hungry. If I get on the scales and I've lost two pounds, I'm hungry! If I've gained two pounds, I get depressed and I'm hungry."*

When following the principles we differentiate *true* hunger from eating triggered by conditioned or habitual responses, old unworkable beliefs, bathroom scales, past experiences, and past failures. Remember, true hunger is a physical sensation in the body caused by the need for food. Appetite is a habitual desire for some gratification, either of the body or the mind, that food won't satisfy even though we think it will. Our physiological hunger is a God-given message in response to a need for nourishment. Our appetite is a result of emotional stimuli, including our false beliefs and tumultuous emotions, that set off our disordered eating behaviors. It is the "lust of the flesh," and it is insatiable: Food will not satisfy it.

Conditioned and Habitual Responses

Consider what activates your unconscious automatic eating. It may surprise you to realize that you have actually conditioned yourself to respond to certain stimuli in a particular way (by eating) and that now, simply by performing the act associated with the stimulus, you set the response in motion. For instance, suppose that whenever you feel lonely and unlovable, you go to the refrigerator and get something to eat. The stimulus is your frustration, rebellion, pain, or discomfort, the response is eating, and the act associated with the stimulus is opening the refrigerator door. You repeat this behavior over time and soon anytime you open the refrigerator door, you feel hungry and you eat. Your response (eating) is occasioned by a stimulus (opening the refrigerator door), an action repeatedly associated with the primary stimulus (feeling lonely and unlovable). Other examples that people in our workshops have shared: The television goes on and out comes the food; pick up a book and pick up the potato chips or peanuts; go to the movies and munch on popcorn; the kids are in bed so it's time to feast; or it's about twelve noon—it's lunch time! Do you begin to get the picture? Conditioned and habitual responses can activate our automatic eating even when we're not hungry.

Old Unworkable Beliefs

We have seen how powerful our beliefs about ourselves can be. We call these "unworkable beliefs" because they don't work for us; they work against us and against the truth of who we are as beloved children of God. Shame, the prevailing sense of worthlessness, leads to beliefs such as I can't change, I am hopeless, or I'm unlovable. These beliefs, based on past experiences, can activate our disordered eating in a variety of ways: You have to clean your plate. Eat three square meals a day. You must include the four food groups at each meal. There is a little bit of dinner left over—too little to save, but too much to throw away. Or, Remember the starving children in Africa. I deserve to reward myself may be a belief based on your having been rewarded with food as a child for courageously enduring a doctor's visit. Or you may adhere to the old rule (now your belief) that a good hostess offers food to a guest and its corollary, a good guest eats what is offered (whether or not he or she is hungry). Many of us believe the lie that food is love, and that offering it or eating it is the same as giving or receiving love.

We may hold unworkable beliefs about our bodies to support or excuse our size, ideas such as: Fat runs in my family, or, I'm big-boned. One woman in our workshop said, "Growing up as a big girl, I always thought I must be big-boned, so I'd eat a lot to maintain my size. But I have an aunt who is overweight, and when she told her doctor, 'I'm big-boned; my whole family is big-boned,' he said, 'Have you ever seen your bones?'" Do you see how easy it would be to conclude that "big-boned" people are doomed to being overweight?

If your eating is controlled by such beliefs rather than true physiological hunger, your eating is probably disordered. Eating for such reasons keeps us mired in the past. Suppose that one of your favorite foods is lasagna, but you believe it's fattening and you should not eat it. Then one day your neighbor brings over freshly baked lasagna! Your reaction is, "I really shouldn't have that," so you rummage around and eat some nonfattening things out of the refrigerator or the cupboard. But what's on your mind? The lasagna—and eventually you end up eating the lasagna on top of everything else. What could you have done? You could have had the lasagna in the first place, eating it from "0" to "5," and you would have been satisfied. Beliefs frequently cause us to react automatically, resulting in compulsive behavior that does not address our actual physiological hunger.

Beliefs like these distort our perception. When you put on a pair of rose-colored glasses, everything looks rosy, doesn't it? After you wear them for a while, you don't notice the rose tint anymore; you just think that's the way the world is. That's how it is with beliefs. If we believe something long enough it becomes our reality, and we never stop to question its validity. For example, where do you think the belief came from that we are to eat three square meals a day? It has certainly been passed on from generation to generation. When people were working out in the fields or on homesteads, they had to expend a great deal of energy in their daily pursuits, and they needed three square meals each day. How many of us today are engaged in hard labor? Not many. For the most part, our lifestyles are more sedentary. Eating habits appropriate for people in those times may not be appropriate for us today. We must examine our beliefs to see if they are still valid and really serve us. In order for our beliefs to serve us, they must be based on present-time truths. Knowledge of the truth informs our will, and we must base our actions on our will, not on beliefs or feelings that may not be aligned with the truth.

Beliefs may become self-fulfilling prophecies. You believe something to be true, you act as if it were true, and sure enough, the predicted result occurs. Both positive and negative beliefs can become self-fulfilling prophecies. Ask yourself this important question: What has it cost you to live life with beliefs that haven't served you? Freedom; self-worth; ability to plan and make wise choices; health; peace of mind; missed opportunities; unfulfilled dreams? When we begin to examine our beliefs and replace the old unworkable ones with appropriate new ones, we can begin to live and eat according to the truth and our new identity in Christ. "Be made new in the attitude of your minds; and . . . put on the new self,

created to be like God in true righteousness and holiness"
(Eph. 4:23–24).

To do this we need to know what our core beliefs are. One way
to find out is to listen to our speech: We can always tell what we
are thinking and what we believe by what comes out of our
mouths. When we label ourselves, we articulate our beliefs. Have
you ever called yourself a "chocoholic" or a "human garbage can"?
Labels can be very powerful; they promote and perpetuate un-
desirable behavior.

I (Judy) grew up in a small town in eastern Oregon where
they had Frosty Freeze ice cream, which I loved. I'd frequently
go and get the largest size possible, so large that they would slide
a straw down the center to keep the mound of scoops from slid-
ing off. My claim to fame was being an ice cream freak. Every
time I would pass an ice cream parlor my friends would say, "Oh,
Judy! We've got to stop and get a cone because you love ice
cream!" And I'd do it, because I had this image I thought I had
to maintain.

That's what labels do. They keep us stuck in a familiar rut. "If
you have been trapped by what you said, ensnared by the words
of your mouth, . . . free yourself like a gazelle from the hand of
the hunter, like a bird from the snare of the fowler" (Prov. 6:2, 5).
Be aware of what you say. Establish new truths about yourself,
consistent with the new identity you have been given in the Lord.

Scales

What happens when you wake up in the morning, step onto
the bathroom scale, and see (arghhh!) that you've gained two
pounds? You decide that your current efforts to lose weight
aren't working, so in your frustration what do you want to do?
EAT! And what happens when you step onto the bathroom scale
and see (yeah!) that you've "lost" a few pounds? What do you
want to do? EAT! You decide to celebrate your victory with a
hot fudge sundae, right? Either way the act of weighing has not
served you.

The scale may be an integral part of the denial/shame/com-
pulsion cycle in your life and can be a powerful trigger for uncon-

scious, automatic eating. Think about how you feel and the games you play when you step onto the scale. Do any of these sound familiar? "It must be broken." "I ate Chinese food last night." "Wait! I'll empty my bladder first." "Maybe if I move it to a different place on the floor or stand toward the back edge." One workshop participant reported that every morning before weighing herself she would wash her face, brush her teeth, empty her bladder, and shave her legs! We'll go to any lengths!

We recommend that you get rid of your bathroom scale. Throw it away! Don't panic and don't worry. In the first place, the scale hasn't really helped you achieve your desired weight, has it? In the second place, your body will tell you whether your weight is going up or down. If getting rid of it altogether seems too radical right now, then consider putting it in the garage or in an obscure place where you won't be tempted to step on it.

Past Experiences and Failures

Past experiences and past failures, particularly dieting failures, also contribute to our fat machinery. How many of your dieting attempts have been failures, maybe even very expensive failures? And what gets activated when we fail? Fat machinery—disordered eating and all of the guilt, shame, depression, and feelings of worthlessness that accompany it.

But far deeper and more profound than our dieting failures are the significant events in our lives that can influence the way we eat. Perhaps the emotions (shame, rage, or pain) that emerge with the memory of a significant event or period in your life activate your unconscious, automatic eating. Food serves as a repressor of emotions, and we may add layers of fat to guard, comfort, protect, or hide ourselves. Those layers of fat are wrapped like grave clothes around the pain, the shame, or the self-contempt associated with all the hurts and disappointments of the past. As we allow our grave clothes to be unwrapped, we are able to identify those experiences and give voice to our emotions. The anger and rage must be addressed along with those feelings of shame and self-contempt so that we can be set free from the past.

"My stepdad sexually abused me," says Vivian. "Then he threatened me and made me promise not to tell. Every night I had to sit across from him at the dinner table. I didn't dare speak: I could see him watching me. So I thought, 'I'll get even with him. I'll eat more than he does.' So I did, until I ended up a size eighteen! This gave me a sense of power over him, that I had conquered him through food, until I began to face the truth and deal with the abuse directly."

> *Food serves as a repressor of emotions, and we may add layers of fat to guard, comfort, protect, or hide ourselves.*

We may be reluctant to deal with the pain of our past, feeling it is too disturbing. We may feel no one would understand. We may feel no one, not even God, was there when we needed help before, so who will help now? There is anger at those who violated or wounded us, anger at God, and probably even anger at ourselves. All of this must be unwrapped and brought to light, but we cannot do this alone. When we take life in our own hands and try to live it day by day in our own strength, we will fail. It is a tremendous burden, one too heavy to bear alone, so we must turn for divine help to the one who can carry it for us: "Surely he has borne our griefs and carried our sorrows" (Isa. 53:4 NKJV).

There are many other stimuli, some quite subtle, that can prompt us to eat when we are not hungry. Some of the common reasons are fear, anger, avoidance, celebration, comfort, reward, it's free—the list goes on and on. When we get down to the bottom of it, however, there is a very powerful belief that acts as the most subtle stimulus of all: I am not worthy of being the size God designed me to be. Now you may say, "That really doesn't apply to me. I've always wanted to be my God-given size." However, wanting to be your natural size and feeling in your soul that you are *worthy* of being your God-given size are two very different things. There will always be countless good reasons to eat when we're not truly hungry, as long as we believe we are not worthy to be the size God designed us to be.

Truth replaces our old beliefs with a new belief. It discards our "good" reasons to eat and brings our eating into present time under the truth of God's Word. When we affirm our fundamental worth and value based on the fact that we are created in the image of God, we begin to establish new beliefs and make way for a prevailing sense of self-worth based on the work of Christ, who has already demonstrated our worth, once and for all, at the cross. "You are worth the Son."[2] "For God so loved the world [that includes you and me] that he gave his one and only Son, that whoever believes in him shall not perish but have eternal life" (John 3:16).

Assured of our worth and value, and knowing that our sins—past, present, and future—are forgiven, our thinking is renewed and we can embrace the self-acceptance God offers us in Christ. We can restate our old unworkable belief—I am not worthy to be the size God designed me to be—as a new belief: I am worthy, by God's grace, to be the size I was designed to be. "We demolish arguments and every pretension that sets itself up against the knowledge of God, and we take captive every thought to make it obedient to Christ" (2 Cor. 10:5). ". . . that you may live a life worthy of the Lord and may please him in every way: bearing fruit in every good work, growing in the knowledge of God, being strengthened with all power according to his glorious might so that you may have great endurance and patience, and joyfully giving thanks to the Father, who has qualified you to share in the inheritance of the saints in the kingdom of light" (Col. 1:10–12).

David Seamands, in his book *Healing for Damaged Emotions* writes, "The healing of low self-worth hinges on a choice only you can make. Will you listen to the enemy as he employs all the lies, the distortions, the put downs, and the hurts of your past to keep you bound by unhealthy feelings and concepts of yourself, or will you take your self-estimate from God?"[3] We need to begin to see ourselves as God sees us: his precious children for whom he sacrificed his only begotten Son.

Observe and Correct—The Grace Principle

The principles for weight mastery are not rules; they are grace-oriented guidelines. Viewing them as such, as a means of experiencing grace, we are corrected rather than condemned by them. By setting up an observation and correction chart for yourself (see page 82), you can monitor your behavior each day and note which of the principles you are applying and which ones you are not. Since we are all flawed, you have permission to be human. There is no perfection in this method, only observation and correction for your mistakes as you go along. Under grace we have the freedom to err, knowing that we are always cleansed by the blood of Christ. This keeps us out of legalism and the distorted thinking that says, *I must eat this; I can't eat that; I did it right, I did it wrong; I was good, I was bad.* Such thinking is part of the diet mentality that keeps us focused outward instead of inward, where the spiritual battle of disordered eating must be won.

A legalistic approach to food, eating, and weight that involves rules and restrictions, right and wrong, good and bad inflames our sinful nature, provokes an all-or-nothing lifestyle, and leads to self-condemnation. It can ensnare us in self-judgment and negative self-evaluations, setting off the litany of self-criticisms that reactivates our old, unworkable beliefs about food and precipitates inappropriate eating in response to stress. Legalistic approaches to weight management treat symptoms only and never address the underlying issues that, while hidden under our grave clothes, continue to control our eating patterns.

A grace-oriented approach, guided by a spirit of love, allows us to observe our behavior and correct it when we recognize that it does not serve our goals or God's purpose for us. Such an approach is forgiving and leaves room for honest self-examination and consistent turning back to God. There is some ambiguity and tension in this process since it requires that we make mature choices, whereas there are no choices on a diet—you're either on it or you're off of it. You either succeed or fail. There is no ambiguity. Observing and correcting requires an active attempt to be attentive to God and to live more fully under his grace.

A grace-oriented approach evokes our body's natural responses on all levels—physical, intellectual, emotional, and spiritual. When we no longer attempt to satisfy our appetites with food and eating and begin listening to our silent hunger, we "make straight in the wilderness a highway for our God" (Isa. 40:3). We allow our bodies, the storehouses of all our past experiences, to be unwrapped, to give voice to the pain, the shame, the rage, and the terror. A grace-oriented approach penetrates the grave clothes and quickens the body with God's healing grace.

A grace-oriented approach is risky precisely because it does evoke our body's natural responses. Many people in our workshops express fears about waiting until their bodies are at a "0." In our experience, that is why "0" is such an important place to begin. Your body will begin to speak to you if you stop keeping it muffled and numbed by stuffing it with food. The emotions will come up, and they will need to be acknowledged and addressed in light of God's glorious grace.

A grace-oriented approach allows us to observe our behavior and correct it when we recognize that it does not serve our goals or God's purpose for us.

Hannah says, "I knew my body was going to speak to me, and I didn't want to hear a thing it had to say. I was comfortable in my head, detached from my body, and I was willing to accept my world the way it was. I knew if my body started to say something I was in big trouble. It all went back to the abuse. Some of that fondling felt good, and being included felt good. Those experiences associated with my body caused me a lot of grief. It was scary to think of getting messages from a body I was afraid to trust."

When we stop eating for all the wrong reasons and follow the principles, waiting for our "0," the body speaks and the desires and intentions of our hearts are revealed. "Through grace, with our assent, our desire begins to be transformed. Energies that once were dedicated simply to relieving ourselves from pain now become dedicated to a larger goodness, more aligned with the true treasure of our hearts."[4] Where once our struggle with food, eating, and weight served as a coping mechanism, a way to survive emotional pain, now as we begin to heal from past hurts we establish a godly sense of our identity and worth and open ourselves to new ways of dealing with feelings and relationships. Then the true miracle occurs. Where once we experienced an unsanctified hunger (our appetite) based on the lust of the flesh, we now begin to experience a sanctified hunger—the hunger for God's love, intimacy, and the transformation of our hearts. Where once we wanted only to lose weight, we now begin to recognize and desire God's greater purpose: not simply to constrain our *doing* (our eating) by the law, but to conform our *being* (our character and the intentions of our hearts) by grace.

As we receive deliverance from our fat machinery, we begin to live freely and not apprehensively. We no longer focus on our obsession with food. We savor the silence, the peace of God's presence. Our lives change from being filled with guilt, worthlessness, and shame to being spontaneous and filled with the fruits of the Spirit—peace, hope, love, and joy. We find our security and significance as God satisfies us with the goodness of his presence. We are restored to our rightful purpose and our true home.

Questions

1. What does the word "deliver" mean?
2. What does the word "freedom" mean?
3. What is "fat machinery"?
4. In your journal list any fat machinery that may have contributed to your disordered eating. Record where each of these habits originated and what you think is the underlying reason for the habit.

Example:

Habit	Source	Reason
I always eat everything on my plate.	Mother	I wanted to please her.

5. What is true hunger?
6. What is appetite?
7. Give examples of conditioned or habitual responses that trigger fat machinery.
   Example: I always head for the refrigerator when I walk into the house.
8. Give examples of unworkable beliefs that trigger fat machinery.
   Example: It's 12 noon so it's time for lunch.
9. What are self-fulfilling prophecies?
10. How has your bathroom scale been part of your fat machinery?
11. In your journal write your understanding of the grace principle of observation and correction.

Scripture to Read

1. Isaiah 53:4–6
*2. John 3:16
3. Colossians 1:10–12
4. 2 Corinthians 10:5
5. Ephesians 4:17–24

*We suggest that you commit this Scripture to memory.

Prayer

Dear God, thank you for your love, which is unconditional and not based on my flawed behavior. I pray that you will give me insight and resolution on whatever is preventing me from overcoming my unworkable habits and ungodly patterns of living. I know you are a gentle God and that you will reveal to me only what I am ready to see. I admit my apprehension as the grave clothes are being removed, but my heart's desire is to be free from the habits that have enslaved me for so long. I am totally dependent upon your mercy and grace and desire only what you have for me. Amen.

Observation and Correction Chart

After each time you eat, place an (X) by the principles you followed. Use one column each time you eat.

Thin Within Principle

1. I ate only when my body was hungry.
2. I ate in a calm environment.
3. I ate while sitting.
4. I ate while relaxed.
5. I ate only the food I enjoy.
6. I paid attention to my food.
7. I ate slowly, savoring each bite.
8. I stopped eating before I was full.

Premenstrual Symptoms (X=Yes, 0=No)

Urge to "stuff"
Headache
Bloating
Craved sweets
Days on menstrual period

Rate the Following (0 to 10)
0=lowest to worst
10=highest to best

Attitude
Energy
Body image
Self-worth
Exercise

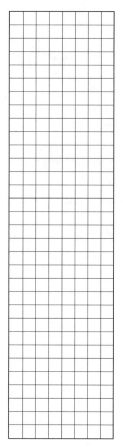
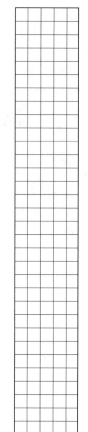
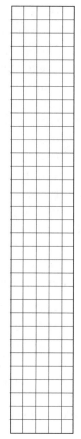

Figure 5

Part 3

Free
to Trust

5

Worth Not Shame

When we accept ourselves for what we are, we decrease
our hunger for power of the acceptance of others because
our self-intimacy reinforces our inner sense of security.
We are no longer preoccupied with being powerful or
popular. We no longer fear criticism because we accept the
reality of our human limitation. Once integrated, we are
less often plagued with the desire to please others because
simply being true to ourselves brings lasting peace. We are
grateful for life and deeply appreciate and love ourselves.

Brennan Manning
The Ragamuffin Gospel

God declares you worthy of love, connection, and intimacy as
his precious children for whom he sacrificed his only son. Your
security, significance, and self-worth are firmly established in this
truth. As his children your need to be valued, cared for, appreciated, and connected to another is rooted and grounded in God's
love.

From birth we have a drive to feel that we are valued. As infants
that drive secures food, comfort, and affection. It is a wordless,
preverbal, God-given need to experience connection, intimacy,

and worth. As we grow, we begin to attach words and images to this need, and we begin to ask that it be met in a variety of ways. God has gifted us with this desire and its proper fulfillment, just as he gifted Adam and Eve in the garden. As they lost their original connection to and dependence on God, we have inherited the loss. Now we are born into families where faulty dynamics may deprive us of the intimacy, security, and significance God intended. Unable to distinguish between the negative messages sent by family members and our own sense of self-worth, we assume that the deficiency lies within us. The result is shame—a feeling that we are defective, valueless creatures who do not deserve the good things in life.

On the other hand, "biblical shame is an appropriate, healthy response when we acknowledge that we are less than God intended us to be and that we are separated from Him by our sin. Although we bear the image of God, sin radically altered our fundamental natures."[1] When we acknowledge this truth, shame is the appropriate response to our true condition. We can then accept with conviction God's gift of grace in Jesus Christ and be transformed. We receive a new identity and a true sense of security and significance. The shame that is rooted in our childhood experiences, however, leaves us with a prevailing sense of worthlessness and insignificance that can lead to the false belief that we are hopeless and cannot change. Our lives then become a quest to prove our worth and to achieve a sense of security and significance by our own efforts. Those of us who struggle with food, eating, and weight may spend our lives performing for acceptance because we equate our self-concept with personal appearance. When our reflection in the mirror is less than perfect we may continue our abusive patterns of starving or stuffing.

If we continue to minimize our self-worth because of shame over our appearance or personality, we are, in effect, criticizing God's unique workmanship. We know God to be the all-wise and all-powerful creator who fashioned us according to his wisdom and power. "Shall what is formed say to him who formed it, 'Why did you make me like this?'" (Rom. 9:20). Are you angry with God for the way he made you? Do you compare and rank your appearance with that of others and with media images? If you do, you are buying a lie and are setting yourself up for suffering. There always will be someone prettier, stronger, or more handsome, and the media images will continue to hold up standards of beauty and perfection that we can never match. Each one of us has aspects of his or her appearance we'd change if we could, but most things about appearance can't be changed. Even if we are strikingly attractive or exceedingly handsome, we may still suffer, living in the constant fear of losing our outer appearance, which has become the basis of our self-worth.

It is a mistake to evaluate our self-worth on the basis of our appearance or performance. Such introspection will merely perpetuate our prevailing sense of worthlessness—our shame. However, if we will be still and let God address our silent hunger, he will graciously show us that he never meant for us to find the fulfillment of our self-worth apart from him. This undeniable, unavoidable longing for a sense of value is a sanctified hunger placed in us by God's design, but we will never experience inner peace until we face the truth that nothing of this world—our appearance, our performance, others' opinions of us, or our past experience—can fulfill our longing for security and significance. Our silent hunger will persist unsatisfied until we can see ourselves not through the eyes of the world but through the eyes of our loving Lord.

> *If we will be still and let God address our silent hunger, he will graciously show us that he never meant for us to find the fulfillment of our self-worth apart from him.*

"Shame often occurs when a failure in our performance, a dissatisfaction with our appearance, or some painful past experience is considered so important that it solidifies a negative self-concept."[2] If we base our view of ourselves on these criteria long enough, we may eventually adopt them as the sole basis of our worth. Then we have (unconsciously) incorporated a lie into our belief system: that we have certain characteristics and flaws that can never be changed. When we take on an identity of shame, we are perpetuating an incorrect view of ourselves and denying God's Word—that we are "fearfully and wonderfully made" (Ps. 139:14). The result of this is that we will appear to the world as nothing more than a reflection of our painful past. If we continue to excuse our failures with an attitude of pessimism and hopelessness, we will never deal with the true self buried under the grave clothes of negativism.

Shame can have a tremendous impact on us if we believe that we can never be different than what we have been. It leaves us feeling trapped and hopeless about ourselves and our future. Because much of what we do is based on our self-concept, our every action will reinforce this negative self-perception.

Sherrie says, "I based my self-worth on my past dieting failures, which resulted from my low self-worth. This produced more failures. It was a never-ending cycle. When I came to understand and accept the unconditional love and acceptance of God, I began to talk more honestly and openly about my feelings without the constant rejection or judgment that were part of my old pessimistic perspective of myself. As I continued in counseling and reading the Word, my sense of self-worth began to change, and I developed a new attitude toward myself and others. I began to see that I could, with God's help, develop a positive relationship with my husband, my mother, and my brother. I stopped feeling hopeless and helpless because of what had happened to me in the past. I stopped pitying myself and feeling victimized. No longer devaluing myself, I was free to reach out to my family in new ways."

Perhaps we find some strange comfort and security in our negative self-evaluation, especially if we place the blame on someone or something apart from ourselves. When we cling to shame and a negative self-concept, we minimize the risk of failure because we rarely extend ourselves. Certainly if we expect little from ourselves, we will seldom be disappointed.

In dysfunctional families where intimacy is distorted or lacking, shame (this prevailing sense of worthlessness) is the usual response. If you were raised in a dysfunctional family, your parents may have sent you the message that you were not pleasing or acceptable to them. Their own shame or lack of self-worth may have been translated into words and actions that instilled shame in the impressionable hearts of their offspring.

Karen related this story: "When I was small, I had a strawberry birthmark on my face. My mother used to tell me, 'You have a face only a mother could love!' It hurt so much! I thought I was ugly and unlovable. Even after it had been removed, she'd see the faint traces and cringe because my face wasn't perfect." Her mother, probably lacking a positive image, passed her shame onto Karen. Karen internalized the message that her self-worth depended on her appearance and her mother's opinion of her. Tragically, children are unable to understand this kind of treatment. "Only as adults do we realize it revealed something sadly missing within the *parents* [or other shamers] rather than something hopelessly flawed within the *children*."[3]

Shame can be activated in a variety of ways: shaming looks, words, gestures, expressions of disappointment, belittling, blaming or accusing, fault-finding, or humiliation. As a small child you may have first experienced shame when your parents got angry with you. Your instinctive, inarticulate response was, "You don't love me anymore!" and your conclusion was that you were bad. If your parents were shamers, they may not have been able to restore the foundation of security and trust by reassuring you of your belovedness. Pressure to perform beyond our developmental level, or shaming of our emotions, can contribute to our prevailing sense of worthlessness. At the core of this identity are the "lies that [taught that] you are the kind of child that deserves disrespectful or dehumanizing treatment."[4] Living with shame you perhaps came to believe that you would never be quite good enough, that the deficiency lay within you. This shame, now internalized, becomes your identity, and is expressed by you against yourself.

Nancy says, "There were days when I couldn't seem to shut off my father's voice telling me I was worthless and would never amount to anything. Listening to that voice I chose jobs that were far below my talents and abilities; I chose relationships that were lacking in intimacy or were even abusive. As God replaced that shaming voice with his loving Word, my life has begun to reflect the fullness and satisfaction he intends me to have."

"[Dysfunctional] shame-based families teach us to avoid the kind of personal disclosure that intimacy demands. Shame tells us that we are 'no good' so we keep others at a distance to avoid being discovered as 'no good' and *rejected*."[5] We experience it as a fear of exposure, a feeling that we don't deserve validation, that at our core we are defective and unlovable. Those who have been abused, humiliated, rejected—denied a place to be comfortable with their own unique identities—are infused with a shame that seems to be stuck in the "on" position. It becomes a steady, throbbing, blaming, nagging source of self-condemnation. As the years pass we are more and more deprived of the intimacy and sense of value we so desperately need, and we attempt to silence our hunger with layer on layer of insulation in the form of addictive, destructive behaviors. As these layers build they gradually become the grave clothes that keep us bound, unable to find the security and significance we long for. An identity of shame and a prevailing sense of worthlessness then influences our feelings and behaviors and leaves us even more susceptible to self-contempt and self-destructive behaviors. This kind of shame prevents intimacy and paralyzes us into isolation. Biblical shame, on the other hand, urges us to repentance, which allows the Holy Spirit to change us from within so we can experience life abundantly, according to God's glorious plan.

Gershen Kaufman, author of *Shame: The Power of Caring,* says that compulsive eating as well as

> bulimia and anorexia are largely disorders of shame. People with those ailments feel at rock bottom that something is wrong with them inside. Sexual and physical abuse are guaranteed by their nature to produce excessive shame, beyond the capacity of the individual to tolerate—anytime the body is violated, that always leaves the person defeated and humiliated.[6]

Shame fuels the belief system that drives our compulsive/addictive behaviors. The false belief that our self-worth is dependent on our appearance, our performance, or others' opinions can only leave us feeling empty and unlovable. Lacking a sense of security and significance (how could God love *me?*), we feel compelled to seek relief in some substance, relationship, or activity. It may be food; it may be sex; it may be an abusive relationship. Our actions (our addictive behaviors) then lead to more shame, and we soon find ourselves in a vicious cycle fueled by and perpetuating shame.

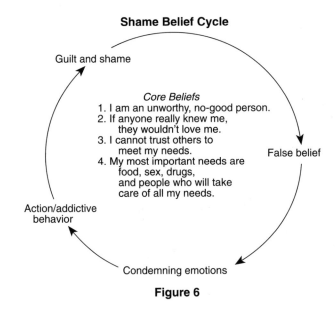

Figure 6

Those of us who struggle with food and eating know this cycle well. We eat when our sense of our unworthiness or unlovability is too much to bear. We eat too much, and then we are ashamed of how much we have eaten or of the consequences of our behavior (weight gain). This results in more self-contempt and shame. So we eat some more. Around and around we go, always ashamed and never satisfied. The remedy for this shame cycle lies in the truth of God's Word.

Truth	**Falsehood**
I am completely forgiven and fully pleasing to God.	I must meet certain standards in order to feel good about myself.
I am totally accepted by God just the way I am.	If I'm not accepted by other people, I must not be acceptable to God.

The truth provides the basis for a new identity and an authentic sense of security and significance. When we accept this new identity, our core beliefs change, our minds are renewed, our emotions and actions change, and the shame/belief cycle is broken.

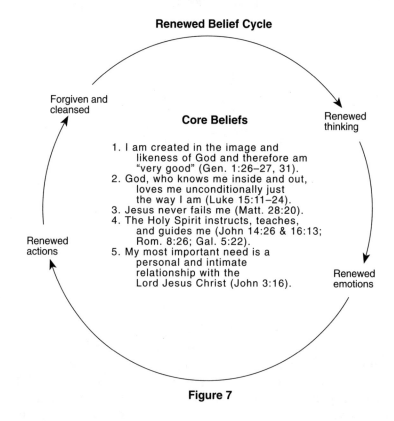

Renewed Belief Cycle

Forgiven and cleansed

Renewed thinking

Core Beliefs

1. I am created in the image and likeness of God and therefore am "very good" (Gen. 1:26–27, 31).
2. God, who knows me inside and out, loves me unconditionally just the way I am (Luke 15:11–24).
3. Jesus never fails me (Matt. 28:20).
4. The Holy Spirit instructs, teaches, and guides me (John 14:26 & 16:13; Rom. 8:26; Gal. 5:22).
5. My most important need is a personal and intimate relationship with the Lord Jesus Christ (John 3:16).

Renewed actions

Renewed emotions

Figure 7

What is the foundation of your self-worth—the false imprints of the world or the truths of the Scriptures? When we know that our value is based on our new identity in Christ, we take on a godly sense of self-worth. With this comes a new direction and purpose in our lives: to live in such a way as to honor the one who laid down his life to give us security and significance.

Guilt

Guilt is not a subject we humans like to address. Yet,

if human beings have sinned (which they have), and if they are responsible for their sins (which they are), then they are guilty before God. Guilt is the logical deduction from the premises of sin and responsibility. We have done wrong, by our own fault, and are therefore liable to bear the just penalty of our wrong-doing.[7]

True guilt is an objective fact, "it is a condition, or state, of being."[8]

"When I was in high school," says Marcia, "I stole money from my mother's purse to buy chocolate bars after school. I rationalized that it wasn't much money and she wouldn't miss it. Now I realize that I was responsible for the choice I made to take her money and I was guilty of wrongdoing."

Psychological guilt, however, is our inner experience, our deep feelings of condemnation, pain, and rejection. The Bible acknowledges legal and theological guilt, but it never tells the Christian to feel psychological guilt.

Comprised of self-inflicted mental punishment, condemnation, rejection, and disesteem, psychological guilt is neither portrayed in Scripture as a positive motivation nor attributed to divine conviction. Even when guilt feelings motivate behavior, they tend to cause repression, depression, rebellion, or other personality dysfunctions. In this way guilt feelings function like the law. They can have no power of positive motivation![9]

Psychological guilt grows out of a shamed identity; objective guilt grows out of an honest evaluation of ourselves. The diagram on the following page illustrates how true guilt, in response to sin, can lead us either through psychological guilt to a self-

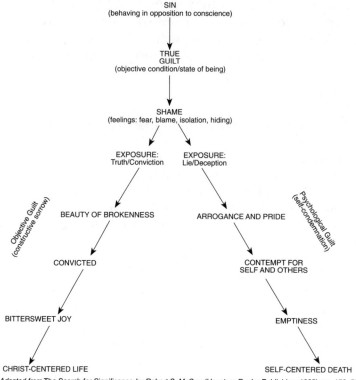

Adapted from The Search for Significance by Robert S. McGee (Houston: Rapha Publishing, 1985), pp. 158–59.

Figure 8

condemning, impenitent response or through an objective pathway to a constructive, repentant response.

Psychological guilt stems from the false belief that we are hopeless and helpless. It results in behavior that further isolates us from the intimacy and love that we all need. We may experience a burden of psychological guilt in our lives resulting from the judgments of others or our failure to behave, think, or look a certain way. We might call it a "worldly" guilt, a failure to conform to the arbitrary standards of others, or guilt resulting from our fear of losing the respect, love, or approval of others. We may bear the burden of psychological guilt for something done to us for which we were not responsible, as in the case of sexual abuse. Certainly much psychological guilt has resulted from our dieting failures or our seemingly substandard appearance.

When this psychological guilt weighs us down and absorbs our attention, it conceals our true guilt and prevents us from receiving what we desire most: forgiveness and acceptance.

> When we wallow in guilt, remorse, and shame over the real or imagined sins of the past, we are disdaining God's gift of grace. Preoccupation with self is always a major component of unhealthy guilt and recrimination. It stirs our emotions, churning in self-destructive ways, closes us in upon the mighty citadel of self, leads to depression and despair and preempts the presence of a compassionate God.[10]

Objective guilt comes from seeing ourselves as we really are— imperfect and sinful, separated from God. "There is no one righteous, not even one; there is no one who understands, no one who seeks God . . . there is no one who does good, not even one" (Rom. 3:10–12). It begins when "the concrete remorse of a particular deed, or a particular false attitude, or a failure for which we feel responsible despite all mitigating circumstances, suddenly presents our human misery . . . as a state of guilt before the holiness of God."[11]

Our capacity to reflect on our own sins and character defects as the present causes of shame allows us to go beyond shame to a sense of true conviction. Acknowledging this true guilt before God becomes the basis for reconciliation and reformation of our character and identity in Christ. Our humility and repentance invokes God's grace and forgiveness, restoring us to a right relationship with him.

If we are responsible in the present for our sin, then "the pain of the past abuse does not justify unloving self-protection in the present," writes Dan Allender in *The Wounded Heart.*[12] When we are ready to accept this mature premise of faith, we begin to see that sin includes our continuing use of food as a way of protecting ourselves. Using food for self-protection, comfort, or as a means of avoiding hurt and involvement is not only an inappropriate way to dull pain, but it is also sin because we have substituted a dependence on food for dependence on God. As we continue to allow our grave clothes to be unwrapped, we receive forgiveness, cleansing, and reconciliation. "If we confess our sins, he is faithful and just, and will forgive our sins and cleanse us from all unrighteousness" (1 John 1:9 RSV). God establishes our new identity in Christ, and we are endowed with an authentic , sense of security and significance.

Using food to dull the pain is sin because we have substituted a dependence on food for dependence on God.

There is no remedy for the gravity of our condition if we fail to acknowledge the extent of our sin, our responsibility, and therefore our guilt. We may be truly guilty of a "refusal to develop, to assume full selfhood or total responsibility in a given situation," says Paul Tournier. This guilt is often reflected in our struggles with food, eating, and weight. "The only true guilt," Tournier continues, "is not to depend on God, and on God alone."[13] Jesus said that of all the commandments, this is the most important: "Love the Lord your God with all your heart and with all your soul and with all your mind and with all your strength" (Mark 12:30). Have you loved food more than God? Have you relied on food, rather than God, to defend, comfort, and provide for your heart and soul? Have you faced the pain of the past (or the present) by asking food, not God, to walk with you through the valley of the shadow? Have you forsaken God when, adopting legalistic diets or other self-controlling measures, you have sought to solve your problems in your own strength?

When we have turned to food instead of God, we have renounced our dependence on God. We must admit our guilt—that we have failed to love God with all our heart, soul, mind, and strength. We must always remember that even when we have failed, we are loved. God calls to us and invites us into a new relationship.

"When Jesus reached the spot, he looked up and said to him, 'Zacchaeus, come down immediately. I must stay at your house today.' So he came down at once and welcomed him gladly.

All the people saw this and began to mutter, 'He has gone to be the guest of a sinner'" (Luke 19:5–7). Brennan Manning, in his book *The Ragamuffin Gospel,* reminds us of the story of Zacchaeus and then quotes this delightful segment from Albert Nolan's book *Jesus Before Christianity:*

> It would be impossible to overestimate the impact these meals must have had upon the poor and the sinners. By accepting them as friends and equals Jesus had taken away their shame, humiliation, and guilt. By showing them that they mattered to him as people he gave them a sense of dignity and released them from their old captivity.[14]

Like Zacchaeus, we're up a tree, fumbling for a foothold in the branches of our false beliefs about ourselves, our vision of our Lord obscured by the foliage of our shame and our sense that we are unworthy to approach him. But Jesus calls us to himself. We are accepted, and in that acceptance comes release from captivity to our shame, humiliation, and false guilt.

"Jesus does not awaken guilt in order to condemn, but to save, for grace is given to him who humbles himself, and becomes aware of his guilt."[15] For guilt, God has given the only solution—the cross on which Christ bore the just penalty for our sins. What happens the moment we trust Christ and his sacrifice? We experience the forgiveness and acceptance available to us through Christ. "Sin is not God's excuse to get rid of us, but the occasion for entering into our lives and setting us free."[16] "Once you were alienated from God and were enemies in your minds because of your evil behavior. But now he has reconciled you by Christ's physical body through death to present you holy in his sight, without blemish and free from accusation" (Col. 1:21–22). Herein rests the antidote to shame. This is not the act of a God who disdains our existence or who counts us as irredeemably flawed. This is the act of a God whose creation is so valuable, so intensely prized, that nothing less than complete self-giving love was and is offered to restore us to his presence.

Beliefs and Our Identity

"Do not conform any longer to the pattern of this world, but be transformed by the renewing of your mind. Then you will be able to test and approve what God's will is—his good, pleasing, and perfect will" (Rom. 12:2). As we have seen, beliefs have a very powerful influence on our eating habits and our identity. To establish a new identity in Christ, we must set aside the false beliefs that determined our old character and actions and enter into our renewed mind. Only then will we experience the renewal of our beliefs, thoughts, and actions and ultimately the transformation of our character. Our goal is to be transformed by the renewing of our minds so that we can discard the fat machinery of the past and establish present-time eating.

Many years ago a group of researchers conducted the Rosenthal study. In it the researchers went into a school, handpicked an instructor, and told her that she would be working with exceptionally gifted children, a group they called "intellectual bloomers." She was thrilled! She had high expectations for their performance, she challenged them, and they excelled. After the study was done, the researchers told the instructor the truth—her pupils were just average children. What happened? She believed they were bright, that belief was transferred to them, they believed it, and, sure enough, they produced. What would have happened had she been told that these same children were slow learners? She would not have expected a lot, and the children would not have achieved much. This study illustrates the obvious: Positive beliefs produce positive results; negative beliefs produce negative results.[17]

What does this have to do with us and with food and eating? First of all, in order for our beliefs to serve us, they must be based on the immutable truth, the Word of God. Knowledge of the truth informs our will, and we must base our actions on our will, not our feelings, because sometimes our feelings may not be aligned with truth. As we base our beliefs on knowledge and our actions on our will, then we experience the power of the Holy Spirit working in our lives.

When you began reading this book, what was your belief about your body? If you had to reduce it to one sentence (I am _____), what would you say? I am fat; I am a compulsive overeater; I am bulimic; I am obsessed with food; I am anorexic? When you believe yourself to be fat, what thoughts and emotions result? Then what do you do? You eat too much, right? Why? Because that's what fat people supposedly do—overeat. The result is, your weight remains the same or increases. What do fat people do when they desperately want to get thin? We've all done it hundreds of times, and we've spent thousands of dollars doing it. We diet. If we do this over an extended period of time, we may achieve a slim body, but what have we accomplished? Our old beliefs are still in place. While our body may look different for a time, our beliefs about ourselves are unchanged, and sure enough, old beliefs eventually take over, we get caught up in eating too much, and the weight comes back—usually more than before. In desperation we find ourselves in search of another diet, and the cycle goes on and on and on.

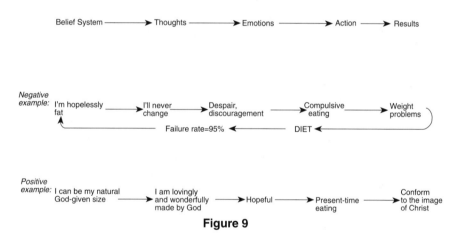

Figure 9

When I (Judy) was bulimic, forty pounds overweight, and very depressed about my life, I managed to pull myself out from under the covers for a weekend outing with some friends on Catalina Island. Unfortunately the weekend festivities came to an abrupt end when I tumbled head over heels down thirty-two stairs and shattered my jaw. They flew me off of the island and took me to the oral surgeon who said, "I have some bad news: We're going to have to wire your jaw shut." I was thrilled! I believed this would resolve my problem permanently. I had previously considered having this done because I was so desperate to lose weight, and here, at last, was the opportunity.

As you know, it is impossible to eat hamburgers and french fries with your jaw wired shut, so my excess forty pounds melted away. I felt great. I thought my problem was solved forever. Four and a half months later the wires came off, and guess what happened? I ate like one possessed and very quickly regained all the weight. Why? Because my belief had not changed one bit since I had not dealt with some deep issues of guilt, shame, and worthlessness, I felt I wasn't worthy of having a healthy slender body.

In order to deal effectively with weight-related issues, it is crucial that we start from a truthful foundation. We must start with our identity in Christ and with a renewed mind—right thinking. "You were taught, with regard to your former way of life, to put off your old self, which is being corrupted by its deceitful desires; to be made new in the attitude of your minds; and to put on the new self, created to be like God in true righteousness and holiness" (Eph. 4:22–24).

Remember, "As he thinks in his heart, so is he" (Prov. 23:7 NKJV). "You will also declare a thing, and it will be established for you; so light will shine on your ways" (Job 22:28 NKJV). When we can truly accept our God-given worth in Christ and base our estimation of ourselves on this truth, our beliefs will conform to the truth. Our thoughts, feelings, will, and actions follow.

You probably know a lot about losing weight if you have done it over and over again, as many of us have. You may even be an expert. That's not what unwrapping the grave clothes is about. In peeling away, layer by layer, your beliefs, experiences, and self-concepts, you will learn to establish a mastery over eating that will serve you for the rest of your life. As you wrestle with your relationship with food in the present, day after day, you need to remember that God has something particular in mind for you where food, eating, and weight are concerned. God is at work in your daily dependence on food, calling you to listen to your silent hunger and to let him satisfy your deepest longing. God calls to us, through the most basic function of our daily life, to look deeply into ourselves, to look beyond a simple change in our size or outer appearance: He wants to transform us from the inside out for eternity.

Our worth and identity are firmly established in these truths: We are created in the image of God; we are redeemed by God; and God's Holy Spirit dwells in us. The God of love and grace puts an end to our self-condemnation, an end to our sense that we are irredeemably flawed and worthless. Our sin and our guilt were removed at the cross of our Lord Jesus Christ, and we have a new identity in him. Are you ready to share at his banquet table and, like Zacchaeus, experience the intimacy, acceptance, and reconciliation that Jesus offers?

A solid sense of your identity and worth is the precursor to your ability to eat and live according to God's intent and to being the person he designed you to be. Teresa, one of our workshop participants put it this way: "I commit faithfully to myself and to God, acknowledging that I am valuable enough in Christ to fill my life with good things—things that please me on *all* levels and that are pleasing to the Lord. Releasing the beliefs that do not reflect God's truth, I also release the excess weight."

With our identity firmly established in Christ, we are free from the shame that fueled our old beliefs and drove our compulsive/addictive behaviors. Free to confess our sin and acknowledge our appropriate shame over our true condition, we can accept with conviction God's gift of grace in Jesus Christ and be transformed. We are blessed with a new identity and a true sense of security and significance. "Therefore, if anyone is in Christ, he is a new creation; the old has gone, the new has come" (2 Cor. 5:17).

Questions

1. Define *shame*.
2. Do you experience a sense of shame over any aspect of your personality, appearance, or past? How does this shame affect your sense of self-worth?
3. How does this shame fuel your belief cycle and drive your compulsive/addictive behaviors? What are the four core beliefs in the shame belief cycle?

4. How does the renewed belief cycle function? What are the five core beliefs included in this cycle?
5. Who was the most dominant person (or persons) in your life when you were growing up?
6. What message did you receive from that person about your worth?
7. What is psychological guilt?
8. What is objective guilt?
9. Upon what truth can you establish new beliefs about yourself to replace your shame-fueled beliefs from the past?

Scripture to Read

1. Psalm 25
*2. Mark 12:30–31
3. Luke 19:1–10
4. Romans 12:1–8
5. 2 Corinthians 5:16–21
6. Colossians 1:21–23
7. 1 John 1:5–10

*We suggest that you commit this Scripture to memory.

Prayer

Dear God, thank you that you desire me to come to you with all of my feelings—the good and the bad. At times I am consumed with feelings of guilt, shame, and worthlessness. I know these feelings are not from you, and I pray that you would help me see myself from your perspective, putting aside all feelings of past failures and worthlessness and letting the truth of your Word renew my mind and fill my heart. Help me to know that I am your beloved, that I am created in your image and am precious in your sight. I pray that you will be at the center of my life and have your way with me as I prayerfully receive your loving-kindness and glorious grace. Amen.

6

Dependence Not Addiction

> The real son of God is at your side. He is beginning to turn you into the same kind of thing as himself. He is beginning, so to speak, to "inject" his kind of life and thought . . . into you; beginning to turn the tin soldier into a live man. The part of you that does not like it is the part that is still tin.
>
> C. S. Lewis
> *Mere Christianity*

It is in our nature to desire to give ourselves over to God's presence in our lives. Our very being cries out for relationship, this rich communion that slakes the thirst of our souls. Our longing originates in creation and cries out for fulfillment in eternity. It is a passion pulsating in our hearts, inspired and nourished by the Spirit of God.

"As the deer pants for streams of water, so my soul pants for you, O God. My soul thirsts for God, for the living God" (Ps. 42:1–2). This passion found consummate expression as God walked with

Adam and Eve in the garden in the cool of the day. Our forebears knew themselves as beloved by and dependent on God, surrendered to and in perfect communion with his will. In this place of unbroken relationship, Adam and Eve "were both naked, and they felt no shame" (Gen. 2:25). Their nakedness bespeaks a face-to-face relationship that brooks no hiding and fears no rejection. This deep and abiding sense of intimacy, security, and fulfillment was based on trust in God's will. Out of his overwhelming love and pleasure in sharing creation with his creatures, God freely met their needs. There was only one thing forbidden to Adam and Eve: "You are free to eat from any tree in the garden; but you must not eat from the tree of the knowledge of good and evil, for when you eat of it you will surely die" (Gen. 2:16–17).

When the serpent beguiled the woman, however, she saw that the fruit was good, pleasing, and desirable (see Gen. 3:6), and so she ate and gave some to her husband also. Grasping for the forbidden fruit, they rejected the position of dependence and ordinariness and attempted to make themselves remarkable, as *gods* (Gen. 3:5) asserting themselves over and against participation in God's will. The fruit was no longer received as a gift given for sustenance and pleasure but grasped as an object of desire, the desire for autonomous existence. They no longer depended on the Creator and Sustainer of all life.

Our souls are indelibly marked by this circumstance. We long to be restored to God's intimate presence—to life dependent upon his will—and yet we put ourselves first, grasping the good, pleasing, and desirable objects of creation for our own gratification. This is our human condition: We put ourselves and our desires at the center instead of God. Our experiences growing up in dysfunctional families, when coupled with the condition of sin, only make matters worse. Yet we are created out of God's love, and as his creation, we long for the taste of the garden— for relationships in which we experience God's delight in and intimacy with us. We are born with a longing to be delighted in, to be appreciated, to be loved, and to enjoy a sense of security and significance.

As children we are wholly dependent on our parents and families to provide for our physical and emotional needs. Because we bear the imprint of God's created order, we trust that our needs will be met out of love. When they are not, or when we are abused or neglected, our God-given need for intimacy, security, and significance is left unfulfilled and our trust is betrayed.

Alexis says, "My father, while not physically abusive, was verbally abusive. He would berate me and call me terrible, degrading names. He would go on and on and wouldn't stop until I was reduced to tears. I never felt safe from his brutal attacks, and I had no idea how to protect myself from him. I would worry constantly about my safety, so I would go overboard trying to protect myself and those I loved. I was afraid to travel; I was afraid my house would be broken into; I was afraid my children would be kidnapped. My life and my world became smaller and smaller as I tried to protect myself. Now I'm certain that God protects me, and I'm much freer to rest in that assurance."

If our authentic need for security and significance is not met, we are left with an ever-increasing silent hunger for love—silent because we are unable or unwilling to express it. In our desperation to satisfy this need we tend to grasp whatever we can in an attempt to make ourselves feel secure, beloved, and worthwhile.

Our authentic need for intimacy, when unmet, opens the door to addictions. The word *addiction* derives from the Latin *addicere* meaning to give assent—to give up or to give over.[1] The very meaning of the word implies surrender and describes the spiritual dilemma of addiction and its hold on the human soul: We give ourselves over to relationships, objects, or substances in our attempt to satisfy our desperate need for security, significance, and love. We may turn to food, performance, relationships, or other compulsive behaviors, and if these provide initial relief, we cling to them, making them the objects of our desire and satisfaction. As these objects become more important, the possibility of addiction grows. When our behavior becomes habitual and we can no longer satisfy or relieve our needs in healthy ways, we become addicted. Addiction results from a misplaced human attempt to satisfy our legitimate, God-given need for intimacy.

Herein lies the greatest risk to our relationship with God. Gerald May writes,

> The objects of our addictions become our false gods. These are what
> we attend to, where we give our time and energy, *instead of love.*
> Addiction, then, displaces and supplants God's love as the source
> and object of our deepest true desire. Spiritually, addiction
> [becomes] a deep-seated form of idolatry.[2]

The addiction itself, rather than God, becomes the driving force
or focus of our lives.

We all substitute self, objects, relationships, or substances for
God. We all commit idolatry countless time each day, but those
of us who come from dysfunctional families move more easily
into intense and binding addictive patterns. Our unfulfilled need
for intimacy and our silent hunger are pushed further and further into our innermost being, progressively buried by layers of
addictive behavior that keep us from experiencing love and intimacy as God intended.

Moving from Addiction to God's Healing

The notion that satisfaction can be found in an object, process,
or substance apart from a relationship with God is the legacy of
the fall. It follows naturally from an attitude of need and ultimately results in a fundamental denial of God's ability to meet
those needs.

When our needs for intimacy, security, and significance are not
met, we are left with a tremendous craving that seems to be self-
centeredness. This apparent self-centeredness is in reality profound neediness. Deeply wounded by our experiences of abuse,
neglect, and familial pain, we attempt to fulfill our need for intimacy with a superficial substitute. Addiction, then, expresses our
woundedness and neediness. If we didn't have authentic unmet
needs, we wouldn't be prone to addiction.

As children, because we could not trust others (such as parents
or families) to meet our legitimate needs, we learned to depend
on ourselves. We became unwilling or afraid to trust anyone, even
God. This lack of trust makes us vulnerable to addiction.

"When I was bulimic," says Rebecca, "and that sense of need
would well up inside me, I felt I had to do something immedi-

ately to make myself feel better. The feeling would overwhelm me, and I would attempt to deal with it by stuffing myself with large quantities of food. I felt I could not let those feelings linger for any period of time. It was too uncomfortable and I was afraid. Slowly I've begun to trust God to comfort me at those tense times. Now I walk through and face those feelings one by one, holding onto God's hand instead of taking things into my own hands. But it hasn't been easy."

In our wounded attempts to satisfy our legitimate cravings, we use food, people, money, objects, and experiences to gratify and serve us. We strive to hold on to these false gods, forgetting that nothing of this world can ultimately satisfy us. Being unable to trust, we *will* our way through life, denying our fundamental dependence on the true God of love, joy, and peace.

Recognizing our wounded condition and our spiritually empty addictions, how do we open ourselves to God's gracious healing? How do we stop grasping for the fruit that we hope will make us feel like gods and yield to a relationship that frees and satisfies us?

In 1975 my dear friend Joy Imboden Overstreet and I (Judy) cofounded Thin Within. Thousands of people attended our workshops, and the organization flourished. Yet with all the success in helping others with their food addictions and by God's grace having overcome my own, I failed to see that I was still an addicted, compulsive person. I had merely traded one addiction (food) for another (workaholism). Thin Within was my life and I served it seven days a week. Work was my passion, my partner, my identity. It was what I turned to for fulfillment and satisfaction. I kept so busy that I wasn't aware of my deepest need—the silent hunger of my soul for genuine intimacy. I was hungry for God's sustaining love, but I was looking for him in all the wrong places. Fortunately God, in his infinite wisdom, loved me too much to allow me to settle for a counterfeit life.

At this point our marketing director, a lovely woman who had a personal relationship with the Lord, recognized that my need was to know Jesus. She led me into the Word and introduced me to the truth that had eluded me for so many years. My silent hunger began to be satisfied as I studied the Scriptures and learned about the person and claims of Jesus Christ.

Because of financial mismanagement, Thin Within unexpectedly collapsed in bankruptcy in 1982, leaving the focus of my existence, my reason for being, in shambles. I felt as if I had been dropped into a dark hole from which I could see no escape. Without Thin Within who would I be? What would I do? My sense of identity and self-worth were wrapped up in my work. Something that I considered so worthwhile had, in fact, become my grave clothes.

> *My silent hunger began to be satisfied as I studied the Scriptures and learned about the person and claims of Jesus Christ.*

One night, having reached the end of my resources, I went to my knees, confessed my sins of self-sufficiency, and asked Jesus to be my Lord and Savior. I asked him to resurrect something out of the mess I had made of my life. He met me there and has since shaped and molded me in the hot fires of life. The process of having my grave clothes removed has been extremely painful, and it is far from complete. Yet he in his faithfulness has restored to me "the years that the swarming locust has eaten" (Joel 2:25 NKJV), salvaging a remnant of Thin Within and turning it into a ministry with him at the center. As Paul says in Philippians 3:8b, "I consider them rubbish that I may gain Christ."

As we erect our idols, whatever they may be, we struggle to stay at the center of everything by controlling people, managing on our own strength, and believing that we are in charge. We think we can do anything through willpower, even control our addictions. But the blessed gift of addiction is that it fails us. If we are honest we eventually reach a point in our lives where we must admit we've lost control. God first allows us to see the futility of placing our hope and trust in the false idols we embrace. Then he invites us to discover the aching, unfulfilled emptiness at the core of our being and to take the first step toward God-centered healing.

Lisa says, "That's what happened to me when I finally allowed myself to hit '0.' Food had always been my friend and companion—it was the one dependable relationship I had. By following the Thin Within principles I finally realized what I had thought was hunger was really my need for companionship. Getting to '0' allowed me to see that the food was a substitute relationship. Then I had to ask, not *what* will fill that void, but *who* can, and will, sustain me? The answer was, of course, our living God."

Suffering and Character Building

"The only goodness in [addictions] is that they can defeat our pride and lead us to more openness to grace."[3] Our pride is often defeated by suffering. It may take a tremendous shock, an experience of hitting bottom as I did when Thin Within collapsed, to dispel the illusion that our lives are perfectly managed, under control, and all together. The pain that shatters our illusion may be the measure necessary to destroy the idols of our dependencies. It may be necessary to reveal the magnitude of our silent, aching, hunger.

"Not that suffering (which is an evil)," Paul Tournier reminds us, "is the *cause* of growth; but it is its *occasion*."[4] What we do when we reach this point of suffering will either result in more pain or unspeakable joy. We can either become *bitter* toward life as we see it or become *better* when we turn to the one who can make us whole. Then suffering becomes an opportunity for grace. "Consider it pure joy, my brothers, whenever you face trials of many kinds, because you know that the testing of your faith develops perseverance. Perseverance must finish its work so that you may be mature and complete, not lacking anything" (James 1:2–4).

God desires that we be shaped and molded into the image of Christ as whole people, not lacking anything. Yet, in our woundedness, we often defend ourselves against anything or anyone (including God) we perceive to be attacking the false yet fragile self we have worked so hard to create. God invites us to release this false self and to receive new life, trusting and depending on his loving will. He wants to take our struggles with food, eating, and weight, struggles that have been the "thorns in our flesh," and use them for our good—to shape and mold our character, to bring us to new life and freedom.

Had I (Judy) not had an eating disorder, I think I would have gone on living in the false belief that I could take care of everything by simply working harder and harder. Through my disordered eating and workaholism, God showed me that all my attempts to look good on the outside couldn't compensate for the flaws and imperfections on the inside. The disordered eating and the subsequent collapse of Thin Within revealed an internal wound so deep and so filled with pain and shame that ultimately I knew I had to look beyond myself for salvation.

Food and eating are so basic that we can't deny their importance in our lives. God, in his infinite wisdom, has shown us our dependency and our need for him in something that is part of our daily lives. If we get a glimpse of what God wants to do with our suffering in this area, we will begin to understand the meaning of the Scripture: "And we know that in all things God works for the good of those who love him, who have been called according to his purpose" (Rom. 8:28). It is a mistake to think that food is an area so insignificant that we should not bother God with our struggle. "I should be able to handle this on my own. Why should God care?" we often think. But God *does* care, and can use this area of suffering as an occasion of sanctification and growth. At the most basic level of our silent hunger, God is there. He is the still, small voice at the center of our chaos—our disordered eating.

Our hope and understanding that God desires to work in this area of our lives makes our suffering bearable. We must be willing to let go, to surrender our will, and to trust God enough to have our grave clothes unwrapped to reveal our true selves. Then we may see how the suffering has served as an opportunity to deepen our faith and to receive God's grace. But our fears often hold us back. "If I take these grave clothes off," Lisa cries, "I will die! I'll feel so vulnerable. There won't be any protection. There won't be any food. I won't recognize myself!"

When our grave clothes are unwrapped, we expose ourselves to insight and revelation. Standing revealed, we will encounter ourselves in a new way, seeing ourselves as God sees us. The purpose of unwrapping the grave clothes is to teach us about our true character. It is here, separated from our accustomed supports and dependencies that we discover how barren our satiated souls really are. When our true nature is exposed, we face the emptiness and silence within our wrappings. Our arrogance and pride are defeated, and we learn what humble dependence on God means. Stripped of our resources and our addictions, we see ourselves with new eyes and are led toward a new response to ourselves, to life, and to God.

Naked, we look on ourselves with new eyes. We experience the possibility of genuine intimacy for the first time. When our addictions were in control, an important, suffering part of us was hidden from the world—a part of ourselves we dared not show. Now that we are not numbing ourselves by gorging, not hiding the truth of the past, not anesthetizing the pain, we are exposed and we are open—open to letting the healing process begin.

When we allow ourselves to be unwrapped, people come closer. No longer isolated by our addictions, we are free to approach life in a new way. We end our protective isolation and risk vulnerability, relationship, and intimacy. When it is just "me and my food," we didn't have to put ourselves out or expose too much. Only when we are stripped of our masks, addictions, and game playing, can we enter into truly intimate relationships, including the restoration of our communion and intimacy with God.

We can then allow God to lead us—we surrender to him. We allow God to feed us—we depend on him. We allow God to give us security—we trust in him. We allow God to teach us—we listen to him. We allow God to love us—we find our true selves in him.

Freed to Depend on God

"Whoever tries to keep his life will lose it, and whoever loses his life will preserve it" (Luke 17:33). When we relinquish control in order to gain our lives in God, he always gives life back to us more abundantly. Dependence—the soul turned toward God, trusting in God, allowing life to unfold according to God's will—centers our lives upon God's grace. It is only then that we experience the profound flow of God's love. It is only then that we can empty ourselves enough to let our silent hunger be filled with all the fullness God desires to give us.

In our struggles with food, eating, and weight we have a precious reminder of our dependence on God. We are dependent on food for life. We must eat over and over again, day after day. God nourishes us daily with the bread necessary to our physical life, and if we let him, he nourishes us daily with the bread of heaven, the presence of his Spirit. Addiction and disordered eating end and dependence begins when we stop relying on our own will to get what we want and begin trusting God to give us what we need. It is then that we will receive and manifest to the world the succulent fruits of the Spirit. When we exchange our weakness for God's strength, our powerlessness for his power, and pray, "Thy will, not my will, be done," we find that the healing love of Christ moves in our midst.

The healing process continues as we put ourselves in a safe environment characterized by ongoing support, honesty, unconditional love, prayer, and the Holy Spirit's love and power. In Thin Within support groups, workshop participants continue to meet and hold each other accountable. The support groups remind us that the basis of this new relationship with food, eating, and our bodies is trust. First, we trust God who created our bodies. Second, we trust our bodies to signal true hunger and to tell us which foods will satisfy us and when we have eaten "0" to "5." In the context of a loving support group, where we are gathered in God's name, we extend that trust to others as we continue to allow our grave clothes to be unwrapped. "For where two or three come together in my name, there am I with them" (Matt. 18:20).

When we begin to trust God, our bodies, ourselves, and the people God has brought into relationship with us, we can let go of striving to gain our life through disordered eating and find our life in God-centered healing. Then "I will say of the Lord, 'He is my refuge and my fortress, my God, in whom I trust. Surely he will save you from the fowler's snare and from the deadly pestilence'" (Ps. 91:2–3). With trust comes honesty, and, as Gerald May says,

honesty before God requires the most fundamental risk of faith we can take; the risk that God is good, that God does love us unconditionally. It is in taking this risk that we discover our dignity. To bring the truth of ourselves, just as we are, to God, just as God is, is the most dignified thing we can do in this life.[5]

We discover our dignity in our dependence on God. As we depend on God and his love, we are freed to live life abundantly.

Questions

1. Define *addiction*.
2. Identify any of your past or present habitual behaviors or addictions.
3. What accounts for your attraction to these addictive behaviors? What would be a more appropriate alternative?
4. How do you feel when you indulge yourself in these behaviors or addictions?
5. How have these tendencies detracted from your life?
6. Give examples in your life when you tend to rely on yourself for strength rather than turn to the Lord.
7. What is the relationship between addiction and idolatry?
8. Identify your grave clothes (if any), why you are wearing them, and what changes you expect when they are removed.

Scripture to Read

1. Psalm 42
2. Proverbs 23:20–21
3. Matthew 18:15–20
4. Acts 26:20
5. Romans 2:1–16
*6. Romans 8:28
7. 1 Corinthians 8:4–13
8. 2 Corinthians 7:8–13
*9. 2 Corinthians 7:10
*10. James 1:2–4
11. James 1:2–8

*We suggest that you commit this Scripture to memory.

Prayer

Dear God, thank you that you, as our sovereign God, control all things. I confess that I tend to take control of my life more than I truly desire. Help me to lay my suffering at the foot of the cross and allow your Holy Spirit to direct my life according to your will. I repent of my compulsive behavior and of substituting a false idol in my life for a living relationship with you. I pray that your will, not my will, be done; that you will be my refuge and my fortress, my God in whom I trust. Amen.

7

The Present
Not the Past

Love is dependent on forgiveness. . . . The extent to
which someone truly loves will be positively correlated to
the degree the person is stunned and silenced by the wonder that his huge debt has been canceled.

Dan Allender
Bold Love

Unwrapping our grave clothes involves resurrecting and resolving the past and being freed from the bondage of old memories,
roles, and feelings. Then we can live unencumbered in the present. The weight we have struggled to release is only a symbol of
the layers of wrappings we've been carrying—the compulsions,
denial, shame, guilt, and old unworkable beliefs and painful past
experiences. As we become aware of our burdensome bindings,
our patient Lord is always near, encouraging us to be unwrapped
as quickly or as slowly as we are able to bear. Layer by layer the
loving hand of the Lord dismantles our crippling defense mech-

anisms and removes the self-protective devices we thought were necessary for survival.

We long to be released from the encumbrances we have been bearing. We want to be set free. "If the Son sets you free, you will be free indeed" (John 8:36). Freedom in Christ is the freedom not to be bound by the pain of past abuse or by inappropriate behavior in the present. Freedom in Christ means living with a renewed mind and a clean heart.

To live an unencumbered life, we must let go of the past, release the victim role, and learn to forgive ourselves, others, and even God. What from your past are you holding on to? We invite you to allow Jesus Christ to accompany you through that painful past, trusting that he will bind up your broken heart and heal your wounds.

Letting Go of the Past

We have seen how powerfully our past experiences shape our beliefs and condition our habitual responses. Long after a traumatic event we may still experience emotional pain. Our bodies may cry out even when our voices are silent, especially if we employ the same coping behaviors in the present we used to protect ourselves in the past. The past, as we are still emotionally invested in it, continues to impinge on our ability to live freely and consciously in the present. The irony is that we think the past has a hold over us when, in fact, *we* may be holding on to the past. We may not have realized that we needed to grieve. We may not have been ready to experience the full impact of a particular painful event. Without this release, we continue to construct our present life around unresolved past circumstances. We may hold on to the false hope that, if we just replay the past often enough or with enough people, we will eventually get what we didn't get.

"On October 28, 1990," says Carol, "my uncle called me at work and told me to go right home. He told me that my son, Rocky, had been in a very bad accident. I hurried home, stunned and scared. When I walked in the house and looked at their faces, I knew that Rocky had been killed. I lost control and started screaming and pounding the walls. I was emotionally and physically in total turmoil. My menstrual period stopped the next day, and I didn't have one for six years. I went to the doctor; he put me on estrogen without success. He's tried everything, but nothing worked. That first year after Rocky died I went down to ninety pounds. I've never weighed ninety pounds in my life! Then, after the shock wore off and I had to face day-to-day life without him, I started eating. I kept getting bigger and bigger, and I didn't even care. I'd wake up in the morning and my first thought would be, *I'm still here.* I kept thinking, *When is it going to end?*

"I've let go of a lot of things during this workshop—things I've held on to for years. I've had to be strong for my mom and for my dad in this tragedy. I haven't been able to deal with my emotions and complete the grieving process. I miss him so much! He's not at home where he's supposed to be, and we can't share the things we used to share. You're not supposed to outlive your children!

"But when we did our forgivenesses in the workshop, I wept tears I didn't know were in me. When I left that night, I felt so unburdened. I released years of stuffed emotions. I can't believe how dead I had felt! I guess I wanted to be dead—my normal bodily cycles even stopped functioning. Now, I feel alive again for the first time in years. I finally let all that grief come spilling out, and what is amazing is that my body responded. I've even begun menstruating again!"

The process of letting go of the past involves grieving. Grief over any loss, or over an abusive or less-than-perfect past takes time. It does not happen according to a schedule, nor does it happen the same way for every person. Yet when we allow ourselves to grieve, we begin the healthy process of growth and change, letting go of the old and making room for the new.

When we let go of our long-time relationship with food, which has become our friend, we grieve tremendously. We grieve the loss of our constant companion. Food was something we could count on and control. Food was the silent partner that would do whatever it was we wanted whenever we wanted it done. We could expect total cooperation. We think we will never be able to replace our companion with one as good, secure, and predictable. So when we let go of that relationship, we experience a profound loss. There is a sense of sorrow that may be expressed with weeping and crying out to God.

All of us involved in struggles with food, eating, and weight began a grieving process many years ago, whether we knew it or not. The first stage of the grief process is *denial*.[1] One layer of our grave clothes is the denied reality of our painful past. Another layer is denial of the extent of our eating disorder. "I used to tell myself that I was overweight because it ran in my family, or that I had big bones. I would never admit that I was overweight because I was overeating," recalls Lisa.

> *When we allow ourselves to grieve, we begin the healthy process of growth and change, letting go of the old and making room for the new.*

Until now, you may have been unable to move beyond that first stage. But now, by acknowledging your desire to have your grave clothes unwrapped and recognizing that your struggles with food, eating, and weight could not be overcome without dealing with the deeper issues below, you took the first step toward letting go and allowing yourself to grieve fully. That simple act was an admission that something, heretofore shadowy and undefined, affected all your choices and reactions in the present. That simple act pierced the silent hunger with a wailing why? That simple act pierced your denial. We may attempt to avoid or postpone confronting the truth about the past by making promises to God, or even by colluding with the entrenched denial of our family system. Maybe you say to yourself, "If they say it didn't happen, then maybe I am imagining it; maybe it really didn't happen. If I just go along with the popular game plan, the feelings will go away."

Once the veil of denial is penetrated, the next stage of grieving begins. You may experience extreme disruption. One person said she felt like she was on a "wild emotional roller-coaster ride." Many emotions may surface, and *anger*, the second stage of the grieving process, will be one of them. Once denial is swept aside, the suppressed anger of many miserable years can and does erupt. As Christine said, "My anger was so out of control it scared me. The rage would appear with no warning. I was afraid I might hurt someone during my uncontrollable outbursts. Now, with God's help, I see that I have a choice—not to react in the old destructive ways when I feel the anger coming on."

When you were a child, it may not have been safe to express your anger. Now, as an adult, you need, or can find, a safe environment in which to allow the anger to speak. While it is legitimate and necessary to experience the anger in the present, the goal is not revenge or abuse of self or another. The goal is to sweep your house clean, to purify your heart so that new life can dwell within you. This may be an appropriate time to find a good Christian counselor or a wise friend who can help you realize and release the full range of your long-suppressed anger.

Stage three is characterized by *bargaining*. Bargaining is tied to the idea that if we just have the perfect body, the grief, the pain, and all our difficulties will be gone. "I thought that if I paid attention to what I ate and controlled myself, then not only would I release the weight, but I would have a perfect life," says Alexis. Bargaining is saying to God, "I'll clean up this part of my life; I'll follow the principles—you take the pain away. Please make it not hurt anymore." Built into bargaining is a time expectation as well. We might feel that we have been doing our part long enough, and we want the payoff now. To our dismay, we may find that God isn't following our timetable.

Depression is the fourth stage of the grieving process. People in our workshops are surprised to recognize the degree of their depression prior to and in the process of releasing their dependency on food. During this stage you may experience the full measure of the loss of food as a friend. This may be a tender time, a time during which you will need companionship, comfort, and guidance. As you feel permission to grieve this loss, you may be assured that this is a sign of health, a sign that you are releasing something you have coveted or have clung to—your old eating habits and your old image of yourself and your world. Robert said, "Before I quit drinking I was a depressed alcoholic. After I quit I was sober but still depressed. It wasn't until I invited Jesus into my life that my depression was replaced by profound joy." Giving up the old self—losing your life in order to find it—is the key to the kingdom and present-time living. It is an integral part of healthy mental and spiritual growth.

Acceptance, the final stage of the grieving process, occurs when we are ready to let go. It comes when we are fully aware of and honest about the past and have made peace with it. Then we are free to embrace a new self-image based on an honest assessment of the past and a willingness to let go of old patterns and beliefs. At this stage we can accept ourselves in light of Christ's acceptance of us and begin building a new foundation for our self-image and choices.

"God has been faithful," reflects Marianne. "Piece by piece he has helped me put the puzzle of my past together. I no longer dismiss my childhood—the pain of the abuse or the disappointment at not being protected. I have acknowledged my rage and deep hurt and have come to see myself *with* my painful experiences and rage, as beloved by God. Now I am able to develop new, loving relationships and express my unique God-given gifts."

We come to this acceptance gradually, not through a forced progression. The stages of grief do not necessarily occur sequentially, and you may progress through them numerous times before you are fully able to let go and accept. In fact, you will repeat the grieving process in large and small ways throughout your life as you continue to shed layer after layer of grave clothes and put on your new identity in Christ.

Grieving, if handled properly, is a healing process leading us to a new freedom: the freedom to accept ourselves as precious jewels in God's crown, to accept the past as it is, and to love others as they are, with passion and generosity. It is by walking through this valley of grief and by dying to the past that we finally let go and accept new life in the present. Christ is with us each step of the way in the power of the Holy Spirit to sustain us, comfort us, and counsel us. Having walked through the valley of the shadow, we receive peace that surpasses all understanding.

Release the Victim Role

It is true that much of our brokenness is rooted in past pain. We may have been traumatized in any number of ways, which in turn fostered low self-esteem, rejection, and even abusive behaviors. Then we, in turn, may have further abused ourselves with our addictive behaviors. It is also true that, until we bring the past to light, we are compelled to repeat those patterns in the present and perpetuate a familiar role—the victim. Our self-image as a victim may be so deeply ingrained that we maintain it by creating situations that victimize us. If we have an investment in remaining the victim, we may exercise control over others by continuing to make them our persecutors, blaming them for our unsatisfactory circumstances, and holding them unforgiven.

"I took a class to enhance my professional ability as a masseuse," says Marianne. "What happened to me in the class was just like what happened to me in school years ago when I was a young overweight girl. If there was an odd number of people in the training class when we chose partners to practice a particular technique, I was the one who ended up without a partner. This was an excruciating experience, and I felt as unwanted and angry as I did when I was twelve years old. I resented the other class members, feeling that professionals should be able to work on anybody without judgments about weight. But in retrospect I realized that I never turned to the person next to me and said, 'Do you want to work together?' I always withdrew in my own wounded way.

"I was tempted to stop going to the class because of what happened. I was ready to throw away something I enjoyed doing because I felt victimized. Instead I went back the next week and tried something new—I asked one of the class members to work with me. To my surprise she was happy to be asked, and I had a great time and learned something new and professionally valuable as well."

When we see the connections between the past and our behaviors and attitudes in the present, we can begin to release the role of a helpless victim. Standing at the threshold of change, we have a choice to make. We can continue blaming parents, or whomever, for our present self-destructive behaviors, our failures, our addictions, or our poor self-image. We can refuse to consider changing ourselves, insisting that other people or situations change first. We can continue to demand that they admit their failings and repent before we feel vindicated and no longer victimized. But in holding others captive, we hold ourselves captive. Our other choice is to allow the healing to continue until we can quit being victims and become liberated victors.

Forgiving Not Forgetting

Forgiving is letting go. When we forgive, we set the offending person free from our demands that *they* change before *we* are willing to change. We set ourselves free from the victim role, old expectations, longings, and unrealistic ideas about what might have been or might yet be.

Much of our shadowy past is littered with the remnants of "deep hurts we never deserved."[2] Some bits may be very old—the pain of childhood sexual abuse, an alcoholic parent, or a parent who deserted us. The pain of this undeserved hurt throbs in us, binds us to the past, and interferes with abundant life in the present. How, in our present life, can we find release from past experiences? God has shown us a way—through forgiveness. Just as Jesus has canceled our debts, now we can release others from theirs. "Forgive us our debts, as we also have forgiven our debtors" (Matt. 6:12). We can forgive as we have been forgiven.

Just what is forgiveness? The definition we use is to cease to feel resentment for, as to forgive an offense; to renounce anger; to grant pardon without harboring resentment. Our simple definition tells us that when we forgive, we cease to feel resentment for an offense. But first we must acknowledge that the offense exists and how deep our resentment runs. We can't begin to forgive until we admit that a grievous wrong was committed—that our painful past and the abuse we suffered is real.

Christlike forgiveness is based on a total commitment to telling the truth. While the biblical model opposes seeking personal vengeance, it does not exclude the appropriate expression of anger.

. . . True forgiveness is not at odds with pointing out clearly who bears the responsibility for a sin.[3]

Hannah describes her experience this way. "For me forgiveness involved, first of all, an honest look at the damage done. I had to acknowledge genuinely how much I had been hurt. That, I think, was the hardest part. You see, I had to stop eating to do that because I masked the pain with food. I ate to stay in my denial. When I stopped my addictive behavior—overeating, sleeping too much, and escaping into books—I was able to get in touch with how miserable I was. When I could focus on the pain and feel how deeply wounded I was, I began to grieve. I wept, I screamed, and I walked and walked. I did whatever I needed to do to motorize that misery—to get my body moving so the feelings could come up and out.

"I had to go deeper into the source of the pain and also acknowledge my part in it—the damage that had been done and how much it had cost me. I had to know who and what to forgive."

Without honesty there can be no real forgiveness, only a gloss of sentimentality over denied truth. Once we honestly acknowledge the extent of the damage and identify clearly who bears the responsibility, we can begin to examine our resentment. Resentment is our bitter hurt and indignation over past pain, abuse, or disappointments, and it is the constant replaying of that resentment that keeps us bound in our grave clothes. Resentment binds us to its object with cords of emotional replay. It is as if we tell ourselves the story, over and over again, in order to keep the familiar struggle alive. Nothing changes. And until we deal with (or resolve) the resentment, we will repeat the same struggle in relationship after relationship, situation after situation.

"I believe," says Hannah, "that when we have extremely strong emotions about someone, as I had toward my dad, we are connected either in a healthy or an unhealthy way. Whether we feel rage, resentment, disappointment, or expectations, we are bound to that person with demands that they satisfy some standard that we put on them.

"Then everyone else who comes into our lives who reminds us of that person gets entangled in those same bindings. The effect is that we cannot have a clean relationship in the present. Because I resented my father for leaving me, I was angry with every other man who came into my life."

Resentment turns our hopes and desires into demands, and perpetuates those expectations and demands in circumstances where it is not appropriate. Binding our present relationships to the unresolved emotions of the past holds us and the other person prisoner, keeps us the victim, and obstructs the possibility of genuine love and intimacy.

Forgiveness, on the other hand, brings about the possibility of creative change. It gives us a way to cut those bindings. Forgiveness refuses to be bound by blame, fault, and revenge. It acknowledges the truth of the offense and admits that a wrong was committed, but it seeks to respond with the creative power of love, out of which arises unforeseen possibilities and new freedoms. Forgiveness cancels our demands and expectations, and empowers us for present-time living and energetic, loving intimacy.

"My husband and I live on a very tight budget," says Gail. "One month our bank balance was seventy dollars less than it should have been. I asked what happened, and he said, 'Oh, the bank must have made a mistake.' I thought that was odd, so I looked in his billfold and found that he had deposited seventy dollars less than the normal deposit. I gave him several opportunities to tell me the truth, but he didn't. In fact, the hole he was digging with his explanations got deeper and deeper. I got more and more angry, concluding that he was a miserable liar, and in my rage I decided to pounce on him and make him pay.

"But by the time I went in for my counseling session I realized I needed another approach. We talked about forgiveness and how to make it safe for him to be honest with me. I went home and after some prayer I couldn't believe the words that came out of my mouth! I was humble, and I am not a humble person. I knew it was the Holy Spirit working in me. The surprise was that my husband melted and told me the truth. He used the money to get a massage. He was afraid to tell me the truth because of my extreme rage in the past. That was an eye-opener! I was able to look beyond his 'lie' and see how my anger had influenced his way of relating to me."

When we are able to step back and be willing to forgive, God gives us eyes to see the fuller picture. Then we can enter into the victimizer's role and see things from his or her perspective.

Forgiveness involves renouncing anger. In order to renounce the anger, we must acknowledge the anger that encompasses the hatred and the hurt we carry with us. Lewis Smedes writes, "When you are wronged, that wrong becomes an indestructible reality of your life. . . . And when you do remember what happened, how can you remember except in anger?"[4] Once we remember, then, and only then, are we ready to embark on this challenging and life-giving process of release and healing. When we forgive, we give up the hatred we've allowed to breed in our heart. We forswear the anger in the sense that we cease nursing it and using it to perpetuate our hatred. Smedes goes on to say that while anger may remain, we lose the "passion of malice." We lose the desire to get revenge on our own terms. We lose the desire to perpetuate our pleasure in drinking from the cup of our own vengeful wrath.

Forgiveness is release. Whom does it release? It releases us from the bondage of the painful past and from the burden of anger, resentment, and repressed guilt. We may ask, do we have to forgive the unforgivable? Yes,

> because without forgiving, we choke off our own joy; we kill our own soul. People carrying hate and resentment can invest themselves so deeply in that resentment that they gradually define themselves in terms of it.
>
> So the longer you wait, the more you risk becoming a person *defined* by your anger, rather than simply a person who has a grievance. The offense and the resultant anger begin to possess you, until your identity is practically demonized by resentment.[5]

We may think we are not able to forgive for the sake of those who have wronged us. After all, why should we let them off the hook when we were the ones violated? But forgiveness is for the sake of the forgiver. As long as we hold on to the feelings and memories, we remain bound to hatred and malice, and our identity is at risk. Until we forgive we will reflect that distorted identity in our countenance or in disordered eating, visible reminders of our spiritual condition. Our calling is to release the guilty person from our demands and allow God to be the final judge and arbiter of justice. As Corrie ten Boom once said, "It is not enough to simply say 'I forgive you.' You must also begin to live it out. That means acting as though their sins, like yours, have been buried in the depths of the deepest sea. The reason your resentments keep coming back is that you keep turning them over in your mind."

There are many reasons we hesitate to forgive, and some of them may be the result of misunderstandings about forgiveness. We may think that forgiveness implies we are condoning the behavior of the offender. Or we may fear that we're saying what happened was really not so bad. But true forgiveness cannot exist without acknowledgment of the extent of the damage. Forgiveness takes seriously the magnitude and the profound effect of the hurtful event. It does not condone the behavior nor does it minimize the damage. Rather, forgiveness honestly confronts the extent of the harm and calls the offender to accountability. "When you forgive, you heal your hate for the person who created that reality. But you do not change the facts. And you do not undo all of their consequences."[6]

Forgiveness is a process rather than a one-time event. Resentment and anger may recede only with time.

We may hesitate to forgive because we think that forgiveness necessarily requires reconciliation—that if we forgive we have to enter back into a relationship with the one who hurt us. This is not necessarily so. Trust requires that both parties acknowledge the truth of the circumstances and come to an agreement about future behavior, and if trust is not restored, it would be unwise to reestablish the relationship. We are *not* called to open ourselves to further harm or abuse. We *are* called to forgive. "Bear with each other and forgive whatever grievances you may have against one another. Forgive as the Lord forgave you" (Col. 3:13).

Another common misunderstanding is that forgiveness means we must forget the incident, that we haven't really forgiven if we haven't forgotten. Forgiving is not forgetting.

> Begin with basics. If you forget, you will not forgive at all. You can never forgive people for things you have forgotten about. You need to forgive precisely because you have not forgotten what someone did; your memory keeps the pain alive long after the actual hurt has stopped. Remembering is your storage of pain. It is *why* you need to be healed in the first place.[7]

Our pain may be released, and we may even be able to wish that person well, but it doesn't necessarily mean that we forget.

> Once we *have* forgiven, however, we get a new freedom to forget. This time forgetting is a sign of health; it is not a trick to avoid spiritual surgery. We have the freedom to forget *because* we have been healed. . . . The test of forgiving lies with healing the lingering pain of the past, not with forgetting that the past ever happened.[8]

Forgiveness is a process rather than a one-time event, and the resentment and anger may recede only with time. "I found that to be true in my life," says Betty. "Someone hurt me very badly and I really wanted revenge. I wanted to hang him out to dry. But I knew that extracting revenge was wrong, and in talking this over with a friend, I decided instead to pray for him. I tell you, that was one of the hardest things I have ever done. I began praying through clenched teeth, 'Lord, I am praying for this so-and-so,' and I was really not too reverent. But gradually my inner attitude began to change, and I must have reflected that change, because that person's attitude toward me changed. You know, I came to the point where I looked at him with a great deal of compassion. I was no longer hurt. But it all began with clenched teeth."

The process is different for every circumstance and can be very difficult, but when we are faithful and persevere in our sincere attempts to follow this bold way of healing, God will guide us every step of the way. "Forgiveness is an interesting process," Hannah reflects. "I am discovering that it is not a once-and-for-all thing. I may make the decision at one point in time, but then I work the process through stages. When new memories come up and I experience a new sense of loss or anger over something, I call to mind my commitment labeled 'I've forgiven him.'"

Once we forgive others, we are ready to take a closer look and begin to accept our part in the drama of offense. "Why do you look at the speck of sawdust in your brother's eye and pay no attention to the plank in your own eye?" (Luke 6:41). "For me, forgiveness has another aspect," continues Hannah, "and that is accepting my own responsibility. Where have I refused reconciliation? Where have I offended? When haven't I seen the good in the other person? When have I harbored bitterness?"

Our unforgiving condition allows us to believe that we have been wronged and stand blameless. One of the reasons we hold so tightly to unforgiveness is that it makes us feel justified. When we forgive, the life we have built on the foundation of our resentment must change. Sometimes we would rather keep things the same, as painful as they may be, than face the immense shift in our perceptions that may prove us wrong. So, we hold our debtors in the prison of our resentment, and the bars are our silent rebuke, our lashing criticism, or our punishing rejection. "If we claim to be without sin, we deceive ourselves and the truth is not in us. If we confess our sins, he is faithful and just and will forgive us our sins and purify us from all unrighteousness" (1 John 1:8–9).

Probably all of us have been in a situation where we have refused to set a prisoner free. When we recognize our part and confess, the surprise comes: "You set a prisoner free, but you discover that the real prisoner was yourself."[9] Then it is as if the response of forgiveness increases in its liberating power. Forgiveness is the desire to extend to another the freedom and release that we ourselves have been given at the cross.

When we remain unforgiving, we give the offenders the power to continue hurting us. "As long as I refused to forgive my father for abandoning me," says Hannah, "every birthday, every Christmas, every special event in my life was a painful experience. Once I forgave him and let go of my expectations, he could no longer hurt me. Afterward I would occasionally receive a birthday or Christmas card from him, and those events became rich and meaningful for me because I had let him off the hook of my demands."

When we forgive, we revoke resentment and revenge and release the pain of our silent hunger. The more we are forgiven, the more we can forgive, and the only way we can be forgiven much is to acknowledge and confess much. Forgiveness springs from a response of love in a heart released by God's love.

Forgiveness opens the door to new possibilities for ourselves and for the offender. When we are not locked into punitive anger or resentment, when we are not blaming and punishing others for our painful past or trying to get someone else to make up for what we never had, we are free to allow God to satisfy our silent hunger in new ways. We are free to embrace the present day and receive present healing. We are free to grow and mature in Christ.

Yet, in the process of forgiving, we will most likely find ourselves wrestling with God. Why did God allow us to be hurt? Where was God in all of our pain?

"You know," reflects Hannah, "for me forgiveness works like this: I forgive them, I receive forgiveness and forgive myself, and then (it sounds sort of arrogant) there is a sense in which I forgive God. Maybe it is not exactly forgiveness, but rather a sense of acceptance: I accept that God allowed all of this to happen and that it is contained in the picture of his perfect love. That is hard to grasp, but he promises that it is true. In the end, I accept that God was involved in this all the way through."

"And we know that in all things God works for the good of those who love him, who have been called according to his purpose" (Rom. 8:28). When we believe in the true sovereignty of God, we are truly free to forgive. Perhaps this is what "forgiving" God really means.

It means that everything we are given to deal with—including ourselves and our psychological material, however intractable—is the result of the creative action of a personal Love, who despises nothing that He has made. We, then, cannot take the risk of despising anything; and any temptation to do so must be attributed to our arrogance, stupidity, or self-love, and recognized as something which distorts our vision of Reality.[10]

The gradual process of forgiveness clarifies our vision of truth and brings us closer to the source of all truth.

Once we have a clearer understanding of what forgiveness involves, we can take the following four steps to forgiveness and freedom:

1. *We begin by agreeing with God.* Jesus says that we are to forgive *not . . . seven times, but seventy times seven* (Matt. 18:22 RSV). In other words, we are called to forgive again and again, and to persevere at forgiving even when we think we are making no progress. This means that we also forgive ourselves as we stumble and pick ourselves up again as we practice the Thin Within principles.

2. *We choose to forgive.* Forgiveness is a choice. It is not based on a feeling but is an act of the will. We may feel like getting revenge and making the offender pay. But getting revenge is neither acceptable nor biblical. We pray to do God's will and let vengeance be the Lord's. "Do not repay anyone for evil. Do not take revenge, my friends, but leave room for God's wrath, for it is written: 'It is mine to avenge; I will repay,' says the Lord" (Rom. 12:17, 19).

3. *We do it.* We make the choice to forgive, and then we act accordingly in faith and obedience. We persevere knowing that forgiveness is a process. Enter into the process (even with clenched teeth) and allow God to direct your will. Your inner attitude will begin to change.

4. *We act out forgiveness and our emotions may follow.* Be willing to pray for the offender. Reach out with a note or a phone call. Search your own mind and heart and remember it is a process that takes time and can only be accomplished by the work of the Holy Spirit within us.

Forgiveness is a provision that God has given us. He knows that we need it and that we will pay a high price without it. Bitterness and malice eat away at our spirit and destroy our ability to walk in love and enjoy true intimacy. So God is serious about our forgiving. "And when you stand praying, if you hold anything against anyone, forgive him, so that your Father in heaven may forgive you your sins" (Mark 11:25). He knows we need to forgive so that we can love and be loved abundantly and intimately.

"Therefore, as God's chosen people, holy and dearly loved, clothe yourselves with compassion, kindness, humility, gentleness and patience. Bear with each other and forgive whatever grievances you may have against one another. Forgive as the Lord forgave you" (Col. 3:12–13).

Forgiveness does not erase the emotional scars or the consequences of real sin committed against us or another, but it does pave the way for real intimacy by freeing us from our grave clothes to "walk in the light [and] have fellowship with one another" (1 John 1:7). It frees us to clothe ourselves with a new identity in Christ.

Feelings and Memories

As we begin to unwrap our grave clothes, we often experience raging emotions and raw feelings that may have their origins in our past. Perhaps these feelings occurred at a stage in our development when we lacked the capacity to identify, understand, or articulate what was going on. The events happened, we grasped on a sensory level the pain, discomfort, or loss, and we registered those sensory experiences deep within our hearts. They are chronicled in our innermost being, and when we begin to deal with the painful past we may experience the hurt again. The emotions that surface can be agonizing and terrifying; certainly they will be uncomfortable. We may wonder how we will survive the turmoil that results.

As we begin to identify these feelings and their sources, put words to them, and express them in a new, mature context, their intensity subsides. When we begin to separate the past from the present and to articulate experiences that, until now, have had no labels, we begin to heal. The process of unwrapping is not just a process whereby we feel the feelings, but a process whereby we identify and put language to them so that they can be communi-

cated to God and others for our development and maturation—
for the work that he wants to complete in us.

"I am an adopted child," says Sherrie, "and I had never seen
my birth mother. I wanted so much to be held, rocked, and com-
forted by her. I thought that if she didn't want me I must be
worthless and unlovable. I used to get headaches and various illnesses in an attempt to get attention and affection from family
members or anyone around me. I wanted proof that I was lovable, and I wanted them to give me what I never got from her.
When I finally found out who my birth mother was and went to
visit her, she cried and told me that when I was born it seemed
impossible to keep and raise a child because she was so young. I
was able to see that her giving me up had nothing to do with not
loving me—it had to do with being unable to care for me and
loving me so much that she gave me to someone who *could* care
for me. Somehow that set me free from the emotional longing
and the manipulative illnesses, and I began to turn more certainly to God to fulfill my sense of belovedness and worth."

Until we are freed from the pain of the past, it can rage and
weep within us, ruling our lives and choices in the present. When
those feelings are strong, they can outweigh our reason, betraying us into making poor choices or giving in to self-destructive,
compulsive behaviors or relationships that continue to enslave
and victimize us. Until we separate past from present we may feel
that we are tossed high and low on the stormy waves of our feelings and that our self-image, our confidence, and even our faith
seems to rise or falter on the swells. How can we "take captive
every thought to make it obedient to Christ" (2 Cor. 10:5)?

We begin by acknowledging our feelings. We can treat them as
little children scattered in confusion around us, and as Christ gathered the children to himself, we can gather our feelings to ourselves. When we ignore or repress our feelings, they do just what
a child in want of attention does: They persist more vigorously
and with greater demands on our time and our mental and emotional resources.

Strong feelings that have their origins in the past usually recur
at times of crisis. At those times we need to be watchful and aware,
ready to receive our feelings in such a way that we bring them to

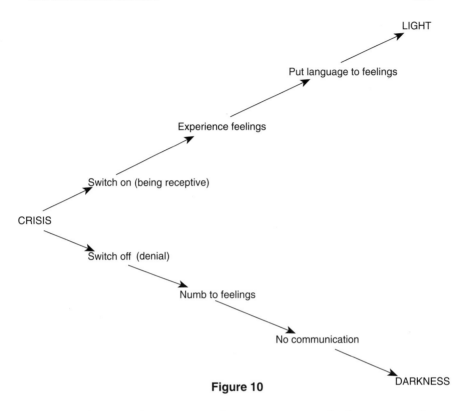

Figure 10

light. "When we learn to put language to our feelings, we take *them* captive rather than letting them seize and enslave *us*. Remember, it takes time to express years of repressed pain."[11] When we do, we render ourselves free to be obedient to Christ.

We can do three simple things when we become aware that our feelings are overwhelming us. First, we can write down our feelings. Second, we can pray about our feelings. Third, we can picture ourselves experiencing our feelings cradled in Jesus' loving embrace. Remember, as overwhelming or as unsavory as our feelings might seem, we are never alone. "Do not be afraid or terrified because of them, for the Lord your God goes with you; he will never leave you nor forsake you" (Deut. 31:6). God will not forsake us as our feelings are brought to light and taken captive— allowed to serve us and God—as we gather them to ourselves in his loving presence.

"Where can I go from your Spirit? Where can I flee from your presence? If I go up to the heavens, you are there; if I make my bed in Sheol, you are there. If I rise on the wings of the dawn, if I settle on the far side of the sea, even there your hand will guide me, your right hand will hold me fast" (Ps. 139:7–10).

> *Sheol* is the Hebrew word, like the Greek word *Hades,* that means "the place of shadows, dimness, half-aliveness, the area of forgotten or dimly remembered." It is an excellent word for our own subconscious selves, where life-forming experiences are forgotten or only dimly, perhaps symbolically, remembered.[12]

When we live an unexamined life, we cannot help but be only half-alive. The place of shadows, the realm of forgotten feelings and memories, encroaches upon our daily lives until we make conscious the unremembered. We have secreted away not only the memories but the accompanying intensity of emotions that as children, we were not equipped to face. When the memory surfaces, the emotional intensity surfaces with it. It is important, at these times, to know God is present and that he will give us the strength to deal with the situation.

"I remember distinctly two incidents when I was sexually molested and only vaguely a third," says Denise. "It is the third incident that holds so many intense emotions. I was so scared. I panicked. I can't force myself to remember everything that happened to me, but I do remember that I was choking and couldn't breathe. I keep coming up against a brick wall in my mind. I want to know the truth so that I can be free—the truth would be easier to deal with than the unknown. But it seems as if I have lost the key that would open the door to this memory. I am ready to face what is on the other side of the door, and I pray that God will help me unlock it."

"But God's love and God's power are not limited by the limits of our memory. . . . God's love is already there. The healing through the incarnate Christ, the embodied love of God, can enter that shadowy pain with full power."[13] While not all memories of past abuse may be brought back to mind, we can still be healed.

The way to unlock the memory is to entrust it to God and his powerful but gentle love. With God's healing light, with a skilled counselor, with trusted friends, and much prayer, the past may gradually unfold. As it unfolds we are released to live unencumbered, available for genuine godly intimacy.

Questions

1. What are you holding on to from your past?
2. Have you grieved a loss related to your food or weight problem? Write about that time in your life.
3. What are the stages of the grieving process?
4. Have you experienced any of these stages? When and how?
5. Define *forgiveness*.
6. Make a list of the people and things you have to forgive.
7. What is resentment? What role has it played in your life?
8. Why do we hesitate to forgive another person?
9. What are the four steps to forgiveness?
10. Write forgiveness phrases regarding the people you identified above. For example: I, _____, out of obedience to God forgive you, _____, for manipulating me with your critical and hurtful comments.
11. How can we take captive every thought and make it obedient to Christ?

Scripture to Read

1. Psalm 139
2. Matthew 6:7–14
3. Matthew 18:21–22
4. Mark 11:25
5. John 8:34–36
*6. Romans 8:28
7. Romans 12:17–21
8. Colossians 3:12–17
9. 1 John 1:7–10

*We suggest that you commit this Scripture to memory.

Prayer

Dear God, I give thanks that you are a mighty God and that your mercies are new every morning. Thank you that you know how heavy my burdens are and that you have asked me to cast my cares on you because your load is light. I confess that I tend to hold on to my burdens even though I know I should give them to you. I confess that I hold on to my anger, bitterness, and resentment, which are eating away at me. I want to forgive the people in the past and present who seem unforgivable, but I can't do it on my own strength. You know that I've tried unsuccessfully to do this. So I pray that you would root out the resentment and bitterness in my heart and free me from the bondage of unforgiveness. I pray that you will give me a clean heart and a right spirit. Amen.

Part 4

Free
to Love

8

Holy Struggle

God, I may fall flat on my face; I may fail until I feel old and beaten and done in. Yet your love for me is changeless. All the music may go out of my life, my private world may shatter to dust. Even so, you will hold me in the palm of your steady hand. No turn in the affairs of my fractured life can baffle you. Satan with all his braggadocio cannot distract you. Nothing can separate me from your measureless love—pain can't, disappointment can't, anguish can't. Yesterday, today, tomorrow can't. Death can't. Life can't. Riots, war, neurosis, disease—none of these, not all of them heaped together can budge the fact that I am dearly loved, completely forgiven, and forever free through Jesus Christ your beloved son.

Ruth Harms Caulkin
Paraphrase of Romans 8

Our silent hunger has at its core a demand that our needs be met. To those of us who struggle with food, eating, and weight, the very presence of the silent hunger is an insistence that we be fed. When we feel and acknowledge the pain and the hunger, we immediately expect food. This is the essence of addictive behavior—turning to the quick fix when the emotions are high, when the pain is throbbing. We try to anesthetize those feelings with food. So, when God says, "Wait," or "Be patient, I am feeding you," often our response is, "Well, great, but it's not what I ordered." We struggle against God's request for patience because everything in us is saying, "No! This hunger doesn't feel good. It hurts and I want to feel better right now! Feed it!" At this critical time we want to put those tattered grave clothes back on.

In this process of unwrapping the grave clothes, the closer we get to the sensitive skin, the more it hurts. The first layers may have been easier, but when we get down near the tender flesh, we want to say, "Stop! This hurts too much." And it is true. After this much unwrapping, we feel like a bundle of raw, hungry demands, and our old nature doesn't want to hurt. We want to continue to take care of our need, pain, loneliness, and hunger on our own. So it becomes a holy struggle simply to choose *not* to put something between ourselves and that pain, between ourselves and another person, between ourselves and God. Holy struggle is choosing to deal with the pain, not to give in to our old addictions and not to develop new ones. We all face this kind of struggle. "I know that nothing good lives in me, that is, in my sinful nature. For I have the desire to do what is good, but I cannot carry it out. For what I do is not the good I want to do; the evil I do not want to do—I keep on doing" (Rom. 7:13–19). This becomes our cry as we engage in holy struggle. We may want to choose new more appropriate behaviors, we may want to satisfy our hunger with good things, but we find ourselves continuing to do the "evil I do not want to do."

"I've replaced food with other things like reading—good reading, instructive reading—still I'm avoiding my life," says Hannah. "I want to belong to people, to engage intimately and transparently in mixed groups, instead, after a speaking engagement, I often retreat to the sanctuary of my own home because it feels safer. How do I begin to make choices that lead me closer to God and more fully into the life I know he wants me to lead?"

Choices: The Old Nature Versus the New Nature

"Those who live according to the sinful nature have their minds set on what that nature desires; but those who live in accordance with the Spirit have their minds set on what the Spirit desires" (Rom. 8:5). When we talk about the old and the new nature, we are talking about two fundamental spiritual realities that influence our beliefs, values, emotions, responses, and choices, whether consciously or unconsciously. The sinful or old nature describes our lives (physical, intellectual, or emotional) estranged from God. It promotes our inclination to deny our dependence on God and to pursue our own desires and old methods of self-control. The old nature is "human nature without God's Spirit, antagonistic to God's Spirit, and acting apart from the Spirit's influence."[1]

The sinful nature seeks to live life apart from God and the guidance of his Spirit. It is the prison of reflexive responses, unworkable beliefs, and addictive behaviors. We may be addicted to food, alcohol, debt, sex, a relationship, or even church activities, if we are seeking to establish our sense of worth or acceptance apart from God. The old nature is characterized by the rigidity of denial (hardness of heart) and deeds done in darkness. It avoids choices because its actions are dictated by events and conditioning from the past. It is reflexive and passive. The old nature is a prisoner of the *law of sin and death* (Rom. 5:2b).

"Those who live in accordance with the Spirit have their minds set on what the Spirit desires" (Rom. 8:5b). The new nature means that our minds are set on what the Spirit desires, when all the inner dispositions, which influence and determine our thoughts, emotions, choices, and behavior, are brought into accord with the Spirit of God. Our new nature in Christ is liberty: liberty from the bondage to food, eating, and weight; liberty from the shackles of the painful past; and liberty from the grave clothes of our addictions. Through his grace we experience the powerful movement of the Spirit from within us, the consequence of the Spirit's authority in our lives. As we stop relying on ourselves and start trusting God, we find that, rather than being controlled by our obsessions with food, eating, and weight, our patterns of sin and addiction *can* be broken.

"I'm not sure what prompted me to turn to anorexic/bulimic behavior," reflects Amy, "but it might have been trying to be the perfect wife, the perfect mother, the perfect daughter-in-law. But when you are my height, five feet eight inches, weighing ninety-three pounds is not healthy. Intellectually, spiritually, and emotionally I knew that was not right. Having had what I feel is a very strong relationship with my Savior from childhood on up, I also knew that what I was doing was a barrier between me and my Lord.

"Even as our family increased to two wonderful sons and two wonderful daughters, I still had this problem. I would binge and purge sometimes three or four times a day. I kept very active: I had a part-time job, and I was a full-time mother; I helped my husband start two companies; I was very active in the church; and all of the time I felt separated from Christ. He was supposed to be the focus of my life, so you can understand the turmoil and guilt that I was experiencing. At one point I was hospitalized for a month. I did have counseling—individual and group therapy—but nothing really seemed to work.

"Fourteen months ago I came to a Thin Within workshop, after praying the night before for the willingness to be open. That's all I prayed for. Thanks to the grace of God, I have not had an episode of binge eating or purging in twenty months. I still sometimes get urges to overeat, and I have gained a few pounds, but the truth is I now look and feel better. I am a little afraid of food from time to time, but that's my old nature wanting to be in control again. Let's face it, I had a pretty bizarre way of controlling my weight for over thirty years, so it is a difficult thing to give up."

You too may experience acute tensions between your old and new nature in your struggles with food, eating, and weight. You may be afraid to let go of the familiar techniques you have used to control your weight, no matter how unhealthy they are, but we know that we are called to walk in newness of life, and that this means putting aside the patterns of dieting, binge eating, and purging associated with our old nature.

The tension between the old nature and the new nature may prompt us simply to try harder to control our actions in order to promote a pattern of behavior in accordance with the Spirit. However, the means toward life in the Spirit is not one of trying harder or of perfection attained through legalistic controls—the means toward new life is *grace*. We observe our behavior and correct it with the compassion of Christ. Remember, you are not only a lovingly and wonderfully made new creation, but you are also in the process of being renewed. Under the authority of the Spirit, your heart lies with Christ and is oriented to Christ. The Spirit enables you to observe, correct, and repent after each fall and to choose time and again for Christ and against your sinful nature.

"Now, I am listening to the Lord," Amy continues. "I have a wonderful support group, and that has been very helpful. I was recently invited to speak at church, and I was open for the first time about my struggle with anorexia/bulimia. Much to my surprise and delight, I found people to be very loving and supportive. I must keep my focus on the Lord, because I am not perfect, but I know that he is working in me little steps at a time. If I am honest, God meets me with his grace as the Spirit has his way with me. Grace is a marvelous gift—it is available to me the moment I turn my will to God's."

Although in this life we are never completely free from the power of sin and addiction, in the process of allowing our grave clothes to be removed, we will experience a distinct difference between the obsolete reflexes of the old nature and the new responses emerging out of our renewed mind, transformed thoughts and behaviors. We still do battle with our old nature. "For the sinful nature desires what is contrary to the Spirit, and the Spirit what is contrary to the sinful nature. They are in conflict with each other, so that you do not do what you want" (Gal. 5:17). We are honest enough to know ourselves to be sinners, and consequently we are no longer willing to be passive accomplices to the old nature working within us. We recognize the tyranny of our old nature that continues to strive for mastery over us, and in the name of Christ and the power of the Spirit we sweep our houses and put them in order knowing that—"the one who is in you is greater than the one who is in the world" (1 John 4:4).

What good is it to be free from sin through Jesus Christ and have every opportunity and every possibility of walking in holiness and in righteousness (with a sense of self-worth, a sense of security and assurance that you are loved by God and valuable to Him) if at the moment of choice you ignore these things and choose to go right on as though you're a slave to sin?[2]

The moment of choice involves the willingness to surrender our old nature to the Spirit of God. Choice engages our will governed by the Spirit. Choice involves examining our old unworkable beliefs and habitual responses and replacing them with truthful beliefs followed by choices that yield action in accordance with the Spirit. "This is love for God: to obey his commands. And his commands are not burdensome, for everyone born of God overcomes the world. This is the victory that has overcome the world, even our faith" (1 John 5:3–4).

Obedient responsibility for our bodies and choosing to eat only when we're hungry and stopping before we're full can be perceived either as an objectionable obligation or as an inviting opportunity. As our grave clothes are removed, we become increasingly aware of the truths God has placed within us: We must not deny our silent hunger; we all yearn for intimacy; and if we allow him he will respond to our needs in all of these areas. When we discover these truths, our surprise blossoms into love for God in return. Love for God shifts our attitude from the objectionable, "I have to avoid it at all costs," to loving response, "It's a choice I want to make," in obedience to him. Since all of this originated from the love of God, our new attitude arises from our deep assurance of God's good will toward us. We come ultimately to the sure knowledge that pursuing godly choices will result in a depth of joy and satisfaction that makes every other pleasure and gratification seem trivial. The basis for our choices then becomes not what will gratify my desire immediately, but what will satisfy my hunger for God and his righteousness. With this silent hunger at the core of our being, we develop a profound desire to respond in obedience to God by honoring our bodies.

Obedience and godly choices are going to come not by our effort or our willpower, but rather by *trusting* God's perfect design for our lives and allowing the Holy Spirit to work within us. As we make choices in agreement with God's will, our awareness of and trust in the love of God grows, and that increased awareness and trust inspires us to choose increasingly in accordance with the Spirit of Christ within us: "Christ in you, the hope of glory" (Col. 1:27).

Making Choices

Nowhere does the matter of obedience and the choice to honor our bodies become so specific and mundane as in our daily struggles with food, eating, and weight. We are graced with the opportunity to exercise, day by day, the practice of governing our conduct by a knowledge of truth and the application of the Thin Within principles rather than by our impulses, desires, emotional pressures, habits, or the whims of the lunch crowd. Our readiness to live a disciplined life, taking our old nature captive to the Spirit of God will determine what, when, and how much we eat.

We are faced with choices every day, particularly choices about whether to continue our addictive patterns. As people set aside for intimacy, given a new sense of security and significance, we choose not to succumb to our addictions but rather to surrender to the will of God. If we set our mind on what the sinful nature desires and respond to that demand, we are going to be grasping and insistent. Surrender implies that we set our mind on the Spirit, being prepared to wait patiently for him to speak to us. It implies that when we become aware of our silent hunger, we let go of the demand that it be instantly gratified with food.

Feeling our hunger and releasing the demand to gratify it leaves us with the hunger sensation alone, uncomplicated by other emotional responses. It leaves us waiting in silence. Then our mind, to fill the void, begins to scan to determine what we've done in the past. We may come up with the conditioned and habitual responses, old unworkable beliefs, and past experiences: "I could go eat a cream puff—that would make me feel better." Then we stop ourselves and think instead, "But I'm surrendering this to God, and I'm learning to wait, so I'll wait and see if I'm at a "0"— if I'm really hungry." So we wait. More feelings arise out of that hunger. Our hunger becomes more insistent! Our mind scans

again. "Well," we say, "I'll go watch TV or read a book," or maybe
we're thinking about food again. Then we stop again and say, "No,
I'm going to choose for now to wait. Maybe as I'm waiting and
listening and thinking I'll go write in my journal or work in the
garden." We choose an alternate activity so that what we've done
in the past no longer has dominion over us. This will allow us
even more time to sort out the feelings that arise and to choose
how to respond rightly. By choosing to stop and not give in to our
disordered eating, we give the Spirit opportunity to speak.

"I used to listen to the voice that says, 'Eat! Eat!'" says Bonnie.
"Now I want to wait and listen to the Spirit speak. When I ask,
'Okay, what do you want from me?' The response usually has
nothing to do with food: Take a walk, pick up a good book, rest
and relax, or trust in me. Those things are really hard for me, but
as I choose to listen and do something other than stuff myself, my
weight problem is being healed."

The sinful nature of our flesh immediately says, "Get the pain
to stop! Get rid of this discomfort! I don't want to feel hungry."
The Spirit says, "Listen to that hunger. Wait for the Lord." As we
do this, we enter a new pattern of behavior in which we are being
continuously renewed in intimacy with the Spirit, choice by
choice. After a while when we don't wait, when we act in a way
that doesn't reflect our new identity, it no longer fits. We begin
to feel like we are wrapping ourselves in old grave clothes and it's
uncomfortable. The addictive patterns, compulsive eating, dieting, bingeing, purging, or anorexia are no longer comfortable and
secure, and they no longer satisfy our hunger for intimacy. So in
each choice we make we find ourselves asking, "Am I responding to the demands of my old nature for some temporary gratification, or in accordance with the Spirit and my desire for permanent intimacy?" This process happens gradually, with the patient,
gentle unfolding of God's will in our lives.

"I've been in counseling for about two years now," says Jen-
nifer, "and until now, I have been significantly overweight. I did
the workshop a couple of times, and I know the principles are
based on truth, so to go someplace else for help regarding my
weight was not an option. But waiting until I'm at a '0' or hungry was difficult for me until I shed more and more of my grave

clothes of resentment and the rage. Yesterday I realized I'd released some more weight and now I see why. Waiting for my '0' suddenly is not so horrendous or objectionable, something that I have to avoid at all costs. I'm ready to embrace it as a good thing. It's a choice I want to make." New choices begin to feel natural.

Choices are the reflection of a renewed relationship with food, eating, and weight. Even if you choose not to eat certain food, which you are *free* to do, choose receiving insight and revelation as you walk hand in hand with the loving God who created you. We cannot have everything, therefore we must choose what we will eat, based on what we hear our bodies tell us and through the leading of the Spirit. These choices are not insignificant, since our physical and emotional well-being are profoundly affected by what we put in our mouths. These decisions are a crucial part of the shaping and molding process by which we become new creations in Christ.

There are five things to consider when making your choice about what and when to eat.[3]

1. *Consider your motivation:* "For the Lord searches every heart and understands every motive behind the thoughts" (1 Chron. 28:9b). Are you at a "0" (in other words, is it really *food* that you need?) or are you trying to satisfy the appetite of your old nature while attempting to avoid dealing with some emotion or conflict? Remember, food eaten for the wrong reason *is deceptive* (see Prov. 20:17). Your choice about what and when to eat is no longer based on your fat machinery, but rather on your renewed mind and your ability to listen to your body and soul in the presence of God. You can satisfy your physiological hunger with food that delights you, but you can satisfy your silent hunger only by turning to God.

"Learning this technique has helped me a great deal," says Denette. "I have tried to satisfy both hungers with food most of my life. I've noticed that when I am starved spiritually, inevitably I end up bingeing on food. Now, as I am in tune with my body, I can distinguish the difference between physiological hunger and my silent hunger for God and make a conscious choice to feed myself accordingly."

2. *Notice the way you think:* "Whatever is true, whatever is noble, whatever is right, whatever is pure, whatever is lovely, whatever

is admirable—if anything is excellent or praiseworthy—think about such things" (Phil. 4:8). Remember, your renewed mind generates renewed thoughts and emotions, which in turn generate new behaviors producing new results: A changed character will be reflected in your body, which in turn will melt down to the size God designed you to be. Most likely, if you are choosing to eat when you are not at a "0," you are engaged in old, negative thought patterns. What unworkable beliefs or conditioned responses are in operation? Once you identify them, you can replace them with thoughts that will generate new results and be in line with your new identity in Christ.

"I have also found it very helpful to visualize my body as if it were a car needing gas," continues Denette. "It doesn't need gas for any other reason than to run efficiently. It has no emotions to fill. I am beginning to treat my body that way too. Once I am satisfied, I stop filling up. I am learning to eat only when I am physically hungry, not for a multitude of other reasons, and this gives me a prevailing sense of peace."

3. *Evaluate your daily lifestyle:* "This is the day that the Lord has made; let us rejoice and be glad in it" (Ps. 118:24). Once you stop being obsessed with food and eating compulsively, you will be surprised how much time you have on your hands! What new things can you do to rejoice in and enrich each day? Make a list of the projects you would like to complete, the activities you would enjoy, the people you would like to befriend or serve, and begin to incorporate those into your daily routine. Find some regular time to exercise in a way that is pleasurable and invigorating. Is there chaos in your daily life? When we slow down and begin to live according to the Spirit, we often recognize how chaotic our lives have been. Perhaps your schedule is so full that you have no time to attend to the important person or event presented to you. Or perhaps your internal emotional state is so frenzied that you keep yourself in perpetual motion to avoid the Spirit prompting you to stillness. It is important to make time available for quiet reflection to appreciate and give thanks to God for the gift of life.

4. *Be vigilant and pray:* "Be self-controlled and alert . . . standing firm in the faith. . . . And the God of all grace, who called you

to his eternal glory in Christ . . . will himself restore you and make you strong" (1 Peter 5:8–10). You are in the process of taking every thought and choice captive to Christ. This involves attentiveness to your old ways of thinking and behaving. It involves a willingness to be honest with yourself and with God as you go to him in prayer. When you invite God to enter your life and allow his will to intervene and govern your attitudes and choices, you will be blessed in all areas of your life—body, mind, and spirit.

5. *Continue to be filled with the Holy Spirit:* "And I will ask the Father, and he will give you another Counselor to be with you forever—the Spirit of truth" (John 14:16–17). We are never left alone and desolate in the grave clothes of our old habits and struggles with food. We may feel alone; however God is always with us, knowing we cannot overcome our struggles with food and weight on our own.

> Addiction cannot be defeated by the human will acting on its own, nor by the human will opting out and turning everything over to divine will. Instead, *the power of grace flows most fully when human will chooses to act in harmony with divine will.* In practical terms this means staying in a situation, being willing to confront it as it is, remaining responsible for the choices we make in response to it, but at the same time turning to God's grace, protection, and guidance as the foundation for one's choices and behavior. It is the difference between *testing* God by avoiding one's responsibilities and *trusting* God as one acts responsibly.
>
> Responsible human freedom thus becomes authentic spiritual surrender, and authentic spiritual surrender is nothing other than responsible human freedom. Here, in the condition of humble dignity, the power of addiction can be overcome.[4]

Reflexive Reactions Versus Reflective Responses

"But Jesus bent down and started to write on the ground with his finger. When they kept on questioning him, he straightened up and said to them, 'If any one of you is without sin, let him be the first to throw a stone at her.' Again he stooped down and wrote on the ground" (John 8:6–8).

Jesus' quiet, deliberate application of truth both convicts the accusers and liberates the accused. It is Jesus' ability to act *reflectively*, not *reflexively*, that reveals truth in the situation and goes to the heart of the conflict between the accuser and the accused. What is the difference between reflexive reactions and reflective responses? The words sound similar, but there is a world of difference in their meanings.

When we are *reflexive* in our reactions, we react impulsively, often without thinking. Often our reflexive reactions are unconscious reactions, arising from patterns established in past relationships and experiences. Perhaps we're not even aware of reacting reflexively. Maybe we wonder why we find ourselves standing in front of the open refrigerator when we intended to take out the garbage.

"I realized I was a bundle of obsolete reflexes," said one workshop participant. When we are wrapped up in our grave clothes, that is just what we are. Numb to our true feelings, insulated from or denying the truth about ourselves, it is very easy for the conditioned and habitual responses dictated by our old nature to kick in automatically when we are confronted with the disturbing circumstances of life.

In the grave clothes of our addictions we react reflexively because of the unresolved pain, hurts, shame, guilt, and unforgiveness of the past. We are attempting to deny the feelings that are raging inside—demanding to be dealt with—by keeping them tightly bound. And we may think we have them under control but in fact we don't. We react reflexively in response to our unresolved yearnings, very much like children having tantrums who cannot express their feelings in a constructive way.

In contrast, when we respond *reflectively*, as Jesus did, we acknowledge and identify our feelings and deal with them honestly. When we respond reflectively we respond authentically to our needs and the needs of another in the present time. We can pause, reflect, stoop down and "write on the ground," and ask the Lord to give us clarity about the root of our reflexive reactions and to inspire reflective responses. Then we open the situation for clear and loving communication. When we come to a place of understanding our feelings, we can respond in a way that expresses our maturity in Christ.

"Now, when I know I am going to find myself in a challenging or difficult situation," says Steve, "I take the time to think the situation through and pray about it. Then I am more likely to make a reflective response and not lash out or react emotionally."

When we come to a place of understanding our feelings, we can respond to others in a way that expresses our maturity in Christ.

Jesus' ability to engage a reflective rather than a reflexive response reveals his ability to enter intimately into the lives of the people around him. His response defines for us an important aspect of the character of a person who is mature and lives intimately with God. One of the greatest characteristics of intimacy is the ability to be reflective and authentically responsive to a person or a given situation. This involves prevailing over our reflexive reactions and applying new, reflective responses born from our new identity and responsive to God's will. When we "are willing to accept full responsibility for our emotional and behavioral reactions in the disturbing circumstances of life . . . realizing that our circumstances aren't the cause of our self-destructive reactions . . . by applying God's truth to those situations,"[5] we can respond reflectively, not reflexively.

When we react reflexively, we are still in bondage. When we are reflective, we surrender and yield to God, allowing him to define our response. Our identity with him defines our character and ultimately our behavior. Surrender means we listen to the hurts, shame, guilt, and unforgiveness and act reflectively. Surrender means we listen for our hunger, waiting for our bodies to give us accurate messages so that we can eat reflectively from "0" to "5." Surrender allows us to take the time to wait for God to speak or for our friend, spouse, or child to help us understand what is really happening emotionally.

"The other night at dinner," says Kate, "I noticed that my son was pushing the food around on his plate, picking at this and that and not eating much of anything. My first reaction was, 'I went to a lot of trouble fixing your dinner and you'd better eat it. You need a good meal after a long day at school!' Of course, he got defensive and angry and said he wasn't hungry. I was ready to make him sit there until he had eaten everything, and then I remembered the Thin Within workshop and the talk about fat machinery. Here I was panicking about my son's not eating dinner because of my belief that we have to eat three square meals a day. So I looked at him. 'Honey,' I said, 'I can see you don't want to eat very much right now. I'm sorry I jumped on you. I forget that you may not feel like eating every time a meal is served. Is there something going on right now that is bothering you?' Well, it turned out there was something going on. If I had persisted with my old reactions, I would have never known what the real problem was. As it turned out we had a good talk, and I learned something about my son's sensitivity that I would have missed had I kept on badgering him to eat when he wasn't hungry."

Our bondage to reacting reflexively can escalate conflict and obstruct communication and the flow of love and grace. We must call on God to lead us into the freedom of responsive, reflective living. When we act out of our new identity in Christ we develop the capacity to listen to ourselves and others, which deepens our capacity for intimacy. This capacity comes out of our ability to be attentive to our emotional responses, reflect on them in light of what we know to be true, and cooperate with God's Spirit in formulating a godly response. This is living a reflective lifestyle.

Those of us who have been on the diet cycle for so many years know what it is like to live reflexively. We may have thought we were living reflectively, because we were living under legalism. After all, didn't we have to reflect on our food choices in accordance with our latest diet? In fact, we were engaging in an all-or-nothing life. Under legalism there is always a sense of deprivation. We are told, "You simply cannot have that," and our immediate reflexive response is to rebel and to want the thing obsessively. That's what diets do. The minute we read the list of what we *can* eat, we start thinking reflexively about what we would *rather* eat.

Under grace we are free to engage our reflective response in setting appropriate boundaries by applying the principles—there is no list. We choose what we want to eat based on our level of hunger and the inner wisdom and discernment we develop as we wait on God. When we don't set appropriate boundaries, we live with the radical swings of our reflexive behavior. Our lives are like pendulums, swinging from one extreme to another. On one extreme, feeling desperate, our old nature kicks in, and we are drawn into the legalism of a radical diet, thinking it is easier to have fixed formulas to follow or someone telling us what and how much to eat. Legalism keeps us as dependent, reflexive children, and as children, we are ready to rebel. When the pendulum swings to the other extreme, we experience wild abandon. We eat whatever and whenever we want without thought for what our body or the Spirit is telling us. We binge; we may purge; we are without boundaries or discipline. Then, in the aftermath of our rebellion, facing an increase in weight or the emotional misery that follows a binge, we give up in discouragement, self-hatred, and despair. Guilt and self-condemnation take over, and the cycle begins again. Both of these self-centered extremes keep us irresponsible and immature, focused on and dependent on the wrong things.

The solution, not necessarily easy, is to surrender to a God-centered life, a life without the extremes of radical dieting or wild abandon. A God-centered life is characterized by reflective attention to the leading of the Holy Spirit, as illustrated on the following page.

Replacing Old Hungers with New Hungers

When an evil spirit comes out of a man, it goes through arid places seeking rest and does not find it. Then it says, "I will return to the house I left." When it arrives, it finds the house unoccupied, swept clean and put in order. Then it goes and takes with it seven other spirits more wicked than itself, and they go in and live there. And the final condition of that man is worse than the first (Matt. 12:43–45).

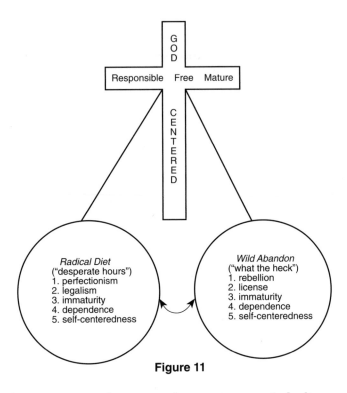

Figure 11

We do not want to leave our house unoccupied after casting out the shreds of our old grave clothes and our haunting hungers. Problems, crises, and old patterns of behavior may push in on us if we allow our swept and clean house to fill up again with such things as resentments, unforgiven past experiences, old memories, and unworkable beliefs. Unless we fill the emptiness left by the departure of our old, addictive behaviors with new hungers for righteous loving, we simply await a greater assault by other habits that can enslave us. Because we are being set free from bondage to our addictive struggles with food, eating, and weight, we are free to be creative and energetic about filling our house with the new projects, relationships, and activities according to the dictates of the Spirit.

We must replace the hungers of our old nature with the hungers of our new nature in Christ. Where our old nature hungers for sin, our new nature hungers for Christlikeness and goodness. We hunger for an honest, intimate relationship with God and those close to us; we hunger to express our sexuality within the framework of marriage, where intimacy can be experienced and deepened; we hunger to express the creative gifts of the Holy Spirit; we hunger to love our neighbor and to serve others; we hunger to care for and enjoy God's created world in new ways; we hunger to respect and care for our bodies by keeping them healthy and toned; we hunger for life in all its fullness. As we experience the joys and delights of life as it is intended, our lustful appetites and preoccupation with food will begin to diminish.

"You know," Jane says, "I had this dogged determination not to give up any of my favorite foods for a long time. I refused to deprive myself of chocolate initially (and still released fifty pounds). But it was only after adopting the Thin Within lifestyle, that I began to lose my desire for chocolate until I was totally delivered from my addiction to it! The wonderful thing about my new lifestyle is that it is not based on deprivation. God changed me from the inside out. The people who told me I had to give up chocolate to lose weight were proven wrong! For me it was important to do it this way, with no extreme restrictions. It is a blessing to know that I could overcome my addictions without being forced into legalism, a way that allows me to be moved by the Spirit knowing that all things come in due time. My old hungers have been replaced with a hunger for God, for letting his purpose for my life shine in and through me, and for ministering to others with conviction."

If we are careful to keep these new hungers satisfied, then we will be far less likely to be enticed to try to numb our old hungers with addictive behaviors that do not truly satisfy. Our goal is not to gratify the cravings of our old nature but to satisfy our true hunger for the love of our living God.

Keeping New Hungers Satisfied

There is no conflict between [satisfaction] of desire and the enhancement of man's pleasure on the one hand, and fulfillment of God's command on the other. . . . The tension that often exists within us between a sense of duty and whole-hearted spontaneity is a tension that arises from sin and a disobedient will. No such tension would have invaded the heart of unfallen man. And the operations of saving grace are directed to the end of removing the tension so that there may be, as there was with man at the beginning, the perfect complementation.[6]

Our new hungers are "the perfect complementation of duty and pleasure, of commandment and love."[7] Our ability and willingness to satisfy these hungers builds a life in the spirit that will support our freedom from disordered eating. How do we cultivate this deep satisfaction of new hungers in our day-to-day lives?

Keeping new hungers satisfied means keeping a balance in our lives. "There is a time for everything, and a season for every activity under heaven. . . . I know that there is nothing better for men than to be happy and do good while they live. That everyone may eat and drink, and find satisfaction in all his toil—this is the gift of God" (Eccles. 3:12–13). For a good part of my (Judy's) life, even after establishing Thin Within, I tended to work very hard, living my life to a significant degree for the gratification and approval I received from others. The only way I could satisfy my real need to care for myself was when my body would literally break down. Then I would find myself in the hospital wondering why my life was out of balance. As I began to examine my activities, I began to see that a holy life, a life lived in service of God and not out of my addictive, approval-seeking tendencies, was a more balanced, healthy life. God is a God of order and he knows that we function best when our lives are lived in accordance with his order. To keep our new hungers satisfied, it is important that the motives of our hearts are pure. Joy and peace will come when we are living for God's glory rather than our own.

God wants our grave clothes removed so that he can resurrect and resolve the old unworkable beliefs, past experiences, and conditioned and habitual responses hidden inside. But, as we are stripped of the very things that formerly insulated and protected us, as we become more transparent, we become more vulnerable. As we begin to experience the feelings we were frightened by or were unwilling to face, we may be tempted to reach for the grave clothes, to slip back into our old, addictive ways of attempting to deal with life by our own strength and on our own terms.

Our holy struggle is to engage life, making new choices, rather than putting our addictions between ourselves and the initial pain and discomfort of living life free of our grave clothes. Our holy struggle is to desire to do what is good and finding ourselves unable, on our own, to carry it out. Holy struggle is to respond reflectively and authentically in present time. Our holy struggle is to admit that, as frightening as it is to be unwrapped, to risk vulnerability, exposure, and transparency in a way that is painful but authentic, only in this condition are we given the possibility of genuine intimacy. Our holy struggle is to surrender to a God-centered life characterized by reflective attention to the leading of the Holy Spirit. And while God knows that our potential for pain is intensified, he also knows that he is bringing us to the threshold for experiencing infinitely more joy. So he challenges us to engage life in a new way, and to effect this he provides us with the spiritual tools we will need to live a life triumphant. The result of our holy struggle is that, with God's help, we will come to experience, perhaps for the first time, the very thing we hunger for—intimacy.

Questions

1. What is the old nature? What is the new nature?
2. Will you ever be free of the power of sin in your life?
3. The freedom of _____ allows us as fallen individuals to do what is right.
4. What two things are important in order to make godly choices to honor our bodies?
5. What disconnects us from the demands of our addictive patterns?
6. What are some alternative behaviors to eating compulsively?
7. What question can you ask yourself to lead you to make the right choices?
8. What five things are you to consider when making a choice about what to eat?

9. What is the difference between *reflexive* reactions and *reflective* responses?
10. What is the solution to living an all-or-nothing life?
11. What does our new nature hunger for?
12. How do we cultivate this deep satisfaction of new hungers in our daily lives?
13. What is the holy struggle?

Scripture to Read

1. Psalm 118
2. Proverbs 20:17
3. Romans 7:14–25
4. Romans 8:5–17
5. Galatians 5:17–26
6. Philippians 4:8–9
7. 1 Peter 5:8–10
8. 1 John 4:4
*9. 1 John 5:3–5

*We suggest that you commit this Scripture to memory.

Prayer

Dear God, thank you that you are a God of grace and that out of your love for me, you have given me freedom of choice. I confess that I struggle daily with desiring to do what is right in your eyes. Oftentimes I take circumstances into my own hands and attempt to force things to go my way rather than have the patience to allow your Spirit to lead me according to your timing and your perfect will. I sincerely desire to live a God-centered life, and I know that to do this I must die to my own selfish desires. I confess that at times I worry that everything about me will be lost in the process, but I see over and over again as I trust in you that your ways are perfect and bring me such joy and peace of mind. Please help me to surrender, and in the process strengthen my faith and trust in you. Amen.

9

Holy Action

Within each of us there is a dark castle with a fierce dragon to guard the gate. The castle contains a lonely self, a self most of us have suppressed, a self we are afraid to show. Instead we present an armored knight—no one is invited inside the castle. The dragon symbolizes our fears and fantasies, the leftover stuff of childhood. When we take the risk and let down the barriers, people respond to us as whole persons and try to communicate with openness and intimacy. Openness brings with it opportunity for a growing relationship, for a wider range of deeply felt experiences. This is the stuff from which friendships are formulated and sustained.

David Smith
The Friendless American Male

When we hear the word *holy,* we may think of something or someone perfect and pure, or that to be holy we must be zealous in our performance of righteous behaviors. Contrary to what our conditioned and habitual thoughts imply, holy action has nothing to do with a set of rules or a system of behavior. It is action distinguishable from any demands that we conform to the stan-

159

dards of the world. Holy action is action set apart by God to develop and increase our capacity for the very intimacy for which our silent hunger longs.

Establishing Holy Action

Our old nature, actions, addictive patterns, obsolete reflexes, old unworkable beliefs, and conditioned and habitual responses interfere with or prevent intimacy. But God shows us a new and very different way for experiencing an abundant life and receiving the very thing for which we hunger. Holy action includes love, knowledge, discernment,[1] responsibility, self-examination, prayer, surrender, and boundaries. These actions increase our capacity for intimacy and establish us in true righteousness and holiness.

Love

"Love is patient, love is kind. It is does not envy, it does not boast, it is not proud. It is not rude, it is not self-seeking, it is not easily angered, it keeps no record of wrongs. Love does not delight in evil but rejoices with the truth. It always protects, always trusts, always hopes, always perseveres" (1 Cor. 13:4–7). If our choices were consistently characterized by the attributes described in this rich passage from Scripture, we could put this book away and apply for sainthood. The reality is that we live up to our high calling and make choices based on love only insofar as we are obedient to God and heed the prompting of the Holy Spirit. The good news is that God, who is Love, *always* fully embodies love's attributes as he acts upon our spirits. So when we come to make a decision, we can apply this verse with full confidence that the perfect love of God acts within us enabling our choices. We can also use this verse as a measure against which our choices are made, asking ourselves how fully each choice reflects love.

Knowledge

"For this very reason, make every effort to add to your faith goodness; and to goodness, knowledge" (2 Peter 1:5). "Grow in the grace and knowledge of our Lord and Savior Jesus Christ" (2 Peter 3:18).

Our choices become more godly as our knowledge of God grows. In order to grow spiritually and to live for Christ we must know God's "good, pleasing and perfect will" (Rom. 12:2). Knowledge of the truth, based on God's Word, informs our minds and leads us to choose to do his *good*, pleasing, and perfect *will*.

We base holy action on knowledge of the truth. We know that the truth of God's Word sets us free. As we replace the old concept of ourselves with truth about our identity, worth, and freedom in God's grace, we are liberated to live an abundant life in the present. We cultivate knowledge as a holy action by spending time reading, meditating on, and studying the Word. Consistent exposure to God's Word informs and renews our minds, feeds our spirits, and frees our bodies from the urge to use food to relieve, comfort, satisfy, or deal with troubling situations.

Discernment

"And this is my prayer: that your love may abound more and more in knowledge and depth of insight, so that you may be able to discern what is best" (Phil. 1:9–10). Love and knowledge lead to discernment. Discernment is a spiritual sense, an ability to perceive or recognize the difference between reflexive reactions and reflective responses that arise from desires corrupted by our addictions and false beliefs. Reflexive reactions arise from our old nature and lead us ever deeper into despair and increasingly desperate attempts to control our lives. Discernment is a God-given sense guiding us and sustaining us in choices that reflect and establish our Christlike character, and it develops more fully in us as we become more intimate with God.

Responsibility

God "blesses us with responsibility and the dignity it contains."[2] "Further, this human responsibility is in the first instance 'not . . . a task, but a gift, . . . not law but grace.' It expresses itself in 'believing, responsive love.'"[3] We do not act responsibly because we must, we act responsibly as a free expression of love in response to the God who is working in our lives. He leads us out of bondage to the wild extremes of our eating habits and into an intimate and balanced walk with him. God calls us, invites us, prompts us to respond to our high calling in Christ, but being a gracious God, he never controls our responses or dictates our choices. In the dignity of responsibility we are free to choose a life of sin or a life conformed to the image of Christ. Responsibility is a reflection of the freedom we have in Christ.

> ### *Responsibility is a reflection of the freedom we have in Christ.*

This gift of responsibility lifts us to our full stature, "the creaturely counterpart of his divine existence,"[4] and lays before us a choice: We can take things into our own hands as we try to control the surge of life's currents, or we can yield responsibly to the Spirit, engaging in holy action out of a God-centered existence, so that we might "guard the good deposit that was entrusted to you—guard it with the help of the Holy Spirit who lives in us" (2 Tim. 1:14).

"To say that somebody 'is not responsible for his actions' is to demean him or her as a human being. It is part of the glory of being human that we are held responsible for our actions."[5] Perhaps this is a new idea to you. Maybe you've seen responsibility not as freedom but as a burden. When we are engaged in our addictive behaviors, the goal is to go numb or to escape life by hiding in the grave clothes of denial, so responsibility seems burdensome. We ask you to look at responsibility from a different perspective—as part of our dignity as God's creation and not as something to be afraid of, misused or abused. We can find true freedom and dignity in exercising our responsibility appropriately.

Self-Examination

"Search me, O God, and know my heart; test me and know my anxious thoughts. See if there is any offensive way in me, and lead me in the way everlasting" (Ps. 139:23–24). Self-examination is another holy action essential to living a righteous and holy life. When we allow God to search our hearts, we allow him to crumble our defensive denial systems. He then allows us to see ourselves clearly, without delusions. Do you really know your weaknesses and strengths? Have you allowed God to reveal your offensive ways?

"When I finally saw that my headaches and physical ailments were my means of manipulating and controlling others," says Sherrie, "I asked God to show me what I really wanted and needed so that I could be honest with my family and friends about my needs for love and connectedness in a way that was appropriate and respectful."

Self-examination, however, is not focused entirely on our weaknesses. God wants to reveal and develop our strengths as well as our gifts, so we can use them as he intends. Only when we see ourselves through God's eyes are we able to live a righteous and holy life, full of the fruits of the Spirit: "love, joy, peace, patience, kindness, goodness, faithfulness, gentleness and self-control" (Gal. 5:22–23).

A searching and fearless assessment of ourselves reveals the areas in which we must be vigilant. Vigilance will help us guard against temptations, which are inevitable. When we are aware of our own vulnerability, we can more easily choose to turn away from relationships, situations, or activities that might arouse our old nature and tempt us in our weakness. "No temptation has seized you except what is common to man. And God is faithful; he will not let you be tempted beyond what you can bear. But when you are tempted, he will also provide a way out so that you can stand up under it" (1 Cor. 10:13).

"After attending the workshop," says Denette, "it was very clear to me how often I ate in response to my hatred for my body. I never liked *me* before. I would look into the mirror each morning and say to myself, *Ugh. Thunder thighs!* The more I said this, the bigger my thighs looked, the worse I would feel, and the more I would want to eat. Of course, that kept me on the binge and diet see-saw. Now I know the solution is to see myself through the eyes of God: to remember that I am lovingly and wonderfully made by him. I know how prone I am to going back to my old habits and thoughts, so I remain vigilant. Frequently I review the principles for weight mastery and allow him to renew my mind and reinforce new habits and beliefs concerning my body and eating."

Prayer

Prayer is the power source of holy action. "True prayer is an awareness of our helpless need and an acknowledgment of divine adequacy."[6] There are two conditions essential for prayer: poverty and honesty. We pray because we recognize our need. If we are self-sufficient and self-willed, believing that we are able to meet all of our own needs, we will never pray. But as we come to God aware of our poverty and honest about the depth of our depravity, we can be assured that God will respond in a loving manner. He is always approachable: he invites us to ask. When we ask, our prayer is "voiced in the imperative mood: . . . give, . . . ask, seek, knock. . . . The request is not a demand. It is a statement of truth, of fact: 'God, I need you.'"[7]

The secret of prayer is understanding the nature of God: he is accessible. When we cry, "Abba, Father!" we acknowledge that he loves us and that it is his nature, as our loving Father, to give. We also have the assurance that he will answer prayer.

> If we are confident of having our needs met when we go to a neighbor in the night; if we are confident that our own father will not give us a snake when we ask for a fish, or a scorpion when we ask for an egg; if earthly fathers who are evil know how to give good gifts to their children; then how much more can we rest assured when we take our requests to a loving, heavenly Father? He who asks, receives. He who seeks, finds. To him who knocks, it shall be opened.[8]

Does this mean we will get everything we ask for? The answer is *no*, but we will get everything we need. In my counseling sessions with individuals who are troubled because their prayers aren't being answered, I use this outline borrowed from an associate:

> If the request is wrong, God says "No."
> If the timing is wrong, God says "Slow."

If you are wrong, God says "Grow."
But if the request is right, the timing right,
and you are right, God says "Go!"

Even the disciples were capable of making wrong requests, requests that were self-serving, shortsighted, and immature. If they were capable of such requests, so are we, although none of us intentionally approaches God with wrong requests.

Two very common prayers are, "Oh, God, please change the other person," or "God, please remove this thorn in my flesh." The motive behind the first prayer is often not a genuine concern for the person but rather simply wanting to get our own way. The second prayer usually stems from our wanting to be bailed out of an uncomfortable or unpleasant situation. This is especially common in those of us who struggle with weight-related issues that aren't resolved according to our timetable. A more appropriate prayer would be: "Help me, Lord. Give me discernment to see what you want to teach me in this situation. Give me the courage and strength to face my own shortcomings rather than focusing on the deficiencies of another or on my own self-will" (see Luke 6:41 and 2 Corinthians 12:7–10).

What if God delays? What if our prayers are not answered according to our timing? God's delays are not necessarily denials. He has reasons for delaying. Sometimes he delays in order to test our faith. Sometimes it is to help us develop character qualities such as endurance, trust, patience, or surrender. Sometimes it is because he wants us to face something in our own lives or our nature that is acting as a barrier or obstacle to our intimate relationship with him.

Prayer that flows from a pure heart is holy action. It is central to a reflective, responsible, and intimate life. Our strength to live such a life comes from meeting God in the silence of prayer. Mother Teresa of Calcutta writes,

If we really want to pray we must first learn to listen, for in the silence of the heart God speaks. And to be able to see that silence we need a clean heart. We cannot put ourselves directly in the presence of God if we do not practice internal and external silence.

Silence gives us a new outlook on everything. We need silence to be able to touch souls. Jesus is always waiting for us in silence. In that silence He will listen to us, there He will speak to our soul, and there we will hear His voice. Interior silence is very difficult but we must make the effort. In silence we will find new energy and true unity. The energy of God will be ours to do all things well.[9]

When we spend time with God, he delights in us, and we begin genuinely to experience delight in him. We find that when we bring our addictive behaviors before God we receive not condemnation but love, understanding, and acceptance, and strength to overcome our weaknesses.

Gerald May writes,

I not only try to pray honestly about my addictions and acknowledge my lack of desire to be free but I also try to turn to God *while* I am engaging in addictive behaviors. Some of my addictive behaviors are not at all the kind of things one would associate with prayer, so turning to God is difficult.[10]

You will be surprised and delighted to experience intimacy and supernatural strength as you surrender to God in prayer.

Surrender

At the heart of holy action is our ability to surrender. It seems paradoxical, doesn't it? We tend to think of surrender as giving up in the expectation that someone else will take over and accomplish for us what we do not want to do for ourselves. Surrender really means that we finally admit that we are absolutely powerless, on our own, to effect any changes in our relationship with food, eating, and weight. Surrender happens when we come to God and place our silent hunger, our rebellion, our reflexive reactions, and even our unresolved problems with food and eating in his hands, admitting that our own efforts have failed us. When we surrender we do not relinquish *responsibility*, we simply stabilize our frenzied experience with the truth: Apart from God, our efforts are in vain. The act of surrender dispels our illusions of self-sufficiency and acknowledges his supreme authority in all areas of our lives.

"Surrender, to me," writes Denette, "means relying on the indwelling of the Holy Spirit and not trying to do things in my own strength. Whenever I try to set my own weight-loss goals and handle my eating problem on my own, I inevitably fail. I have found it essential to rely on the power of the Holy Spirit. It is a continuous process of reminding myself to yield the control to him yet walk responsibly with him.

"When I try to rely on myself, I tend to step back to my old ways. For example, I find it very easy to control my food intake when I'm on vacation, because there is no stress. Also my appetite diminishes when I'm ill. I used to take advantage of these occasions to lose as much weight as possible. When the illness or the vacation ended, I would be thinner, more famished, and more fearful than ever of regaining the weight. This would trigger my feast-or-famine mentality and to avoid gaining weight, I would purge whenever I binged, and the habit would be more firmly ingrained. It is only by yielding to God as I apply the Thin Within principles that I am able to trust him and *not* keep striving to become thinner and thinner. I believe I am now beginning the process of stepping aside from my sinful nature of self-reliance and acting in accordance with the Spirit."

We talk about surrender as holy action because in our struggles with food, eating, and weight we do not give up our illusion of control easily. We must surrender again and again and again, day by day, bite by bite, believing that each time we confront our desire to take back the control, our humble willingness to give it up again is all that God requires.

Boundaries

With holy action comes the development of boundaries.[11] Boundaries are the conditions we establish to maintain our rightful sense of physical and emotional distinction from other people and things in the world around us. A boundary is a line defining the limit of your property. It not only defines who you are but also who you are not. Boundaries also delineate what you are (and what you are not) responsible for. When you establish boundaries, you are exercising your right to set limits and protect yourself. Boundaries define the dignity of your uniquely created self and prevent you from losing your identity by inappropriately adopting the personality or behavior of someone else. Your body is the most basic boundary you have.

Boundaries are always in the service and protection of intimacy. Boundaries protect our treasures: our feelings, attitudes, behaviors, choices, values, limits, talents, thoughts, and intimacy. They help us take appropriate control of these treasures and exercise responsible stewardship over them. Without boundaries we may suffer from depression—a sense of hopelessness and an attitude of despair. We may reengage in our compulsive and addictive behaviors because we have not acquired the ability to stand up and say "no." Without boundaries we may experience problems in relationships if we attempt to exercise inappropriate control over the other person. We may fail to experience intimacy in relationships, if we are unable to ask for what we want and need. We may find ourselves in chaotic relationships because of unclear boundaries, not knowing where we stop and the other person begins. We may find ourselves so worn out from trying to keep everyone happy that we cannot concentrate. We may never reach our goals; we live from crisis to crisis, living in anxiety and dread about the future; we may become aggressive or passive, reacting out of our old reflexes to people and circumstances in our lives.

"However, when we establish appropriate boundaries, we clarify relationships and function appropriately within them. We put into effect the law of sowing and reaping, cause and effect."[12] Boundaries cause the consequences of the sin to fall into the field of that sinner, limiting the consequences of the action to the responsible person. This means you can keep the contamination of another person's sinful actions out of your field by setting a boundary that places the responsibility where it is due. It also means accepting responsibility for your own behaviors, taking the consequences, releasing the victim role and the need to blame.

Boundaries are necessary for healthy relationships, but they must be clearly and verbally communicated to the other person.

Often we communicate our boundaries indirectly or manipulatively—we get headaches, we get sick, or we withdraw. Or we keep putting on the weight that we think defines, separates, or protects us from the rest of the world. For our boundaries to become holy action, they must be active and articulated. A free "no" leads to a free "yes." When we can't say *no,* our *yes* doesn't mean anything. "Simply let your 'yes' be 'yes,' and your 'no' be 'no'" (Matt. 5:37). When you act reflectively and set a clear boundary, you are establishing holy action—you are becoming holy. It is like putting up a fence around a sacred ground to keep abusive people and abusive habits out of your life.

We begin to establish boundaries in our lives by following the principles for weight mastery. The principles are the holy habits at the heart of a life of God-centered responsibility for dealing with our struggles with food, eating, and weight. Applying the principles, we let the Spirit lead so that appropriate boundaries are set from within. We have discovered that within those boundaries we have freedom—freedom to eat the foods we enjoy. Freedom is not wild abandon; we can eat chocolate cake if that's what we enjoy, but we don't eat the *whole* chocolate cake. Under legalism—diets—we attempt to conform to rigid boundaries that have been externally placed on us.

If we have good boundaries, and we are secure in who we are in Christ, we know what to allow in and what to keep out. We know the difference between stuffing and eating "0" to "5." We know when we are satisfied. If we have no boundaries our identity is unclear, and we never know when enough is enough. The things that we allow in and the things we exclude determine our identity, our feelings, attitudes, behaviors, choices, values, limits, talents, thoughts, and love. Our capacity for genuinely intimate relationships with our loving God and his people will be greatly increased if we have set good boundaries. And the result will be that we will *live* life abundantly, according to God's plan.

Living Unwrapped

If we discard our grave clothes, what on earth will happen to us? We all want to look good; we all have a need to make a good showing. The tendency of our old nature is to do whatever (or cover up whatever) we think we must to present ourselves in what we consider to be the most acceptable light. Most of us think that if we reveal our innermost selves, we will be rejected and abandoned, isolated and hungry (again) for intimacy. But the truth is that our grave clothes are the greatest barrier to intimacy. The more we reveal of ourselves—the more vulnerable and transparent we are—the more appealing, attractive, and authentic we become. Instead of exuding the stench of death, we emit the sweet fragrance Christ.

> *The more we reveal of ourselves—*
> *the more vulnerable and transparent we*
> *are—the more appealing, attractive,*
> *and authentic we become.*

Hannah says, "All these years I've told myself that I was managing brilliantly by using my humor and intelligence to keep people at a distance, because I believed that I wasn't worthy of any real intimacy. I considered *distant* intimacy a success. To unwrap my grave clothes, let go of my old beliefs and fears and let people get closer was simultaneously astonishing and terrifying. The astonishing thing was that the more I revealed, the more people really cared about me. And it was terrifying because I realized that I didn't know how to simply be who I am."

All of us have a tendency to think that the parts of us that are lovable are all the external things—our appearance, our skills, our successes. Do you remember the old "Invisible Man" movie? As the bandages came off, there was nothing on the inside. Only the bandages gave him form. We are afraid that when the grave clothes, the external trappings, come off, people will see nothing lovable on the inside. The truth is people are drawn to us when we are willing to reveal our true selves—when we show who we really are and are willing to risk genuine intimacy.

God's purpose is to satisfy our silent hunger for intimacy by unwrapping the grave clothes of our addictions and drawing us into deeper intimacy with himself and others. But we try to satisfy our own needs by taking things into our own hands, just like Adam and Eve. When we can't accomplish this we attempt to numb the pain and protect ourselves with layers of insulation. This describes the spiritual battle we are in.

"I knew that I was going to a battle," says Hannah, "and I knew that I was going to be a casualty. I didn't want to face the struggle that was going on inside of me, so I went numb. To protect myself, I wrapped up in as many layers of grave clothes as I could get my hands on—the comfort of food, avoiding people, turning off my phone, staying away from relationships, manipulating people to keep them at a safe distance. I even insisted that my husband and I move when people got too close.

"But then Christ called me to life, showing me that the only way to win was to fight the battle using his armor. Surrendering to his will has caused me to discard the armor of my own design. He calls me to stay put, to set aside my addictive behaviors, and to present myself naked and defenseless to him, praying for his help. That's when he began to teach me the truth about spiritual armor."

Spiritual Armor

God offers us armor, not the illusory protection of our grave clothes, but the spiritual armor necessary to win our spiritual battle. Now the irony is that our grave clothes, because they are familiar, may feel more substantial than spiritual armor. In fact, our old external armor (our grave clothes) is not sufficient because we do not face an external battle—we face an internal spiritual battle for which we need spiritual armor.

Intimacy requires that we do battle so that the adversary will not have his way with us where food and eating are concerned. It requires that we stand up and receive the fullness of our precious lives in Christ Jesus. In this battle, there is danger and risk, and there is potential for being wounded, but God's provision— the full armor of God—will protect us.

Finally, be strong in the Lord and in his mighty power. Put on the full armor of God, so that when the day of evil comes, you may be able to stand your ground, and after you have done everything, to stand. Stand firm then, with the belt of truth buckled around your waist, with the breastplate of righteousness in place, and with your feet fitted with the readiness that comes from the gospel of peace. In addition to all this, take up the shield of faith, with which you can extinguish all the flaming arrows of the evil one. Take the helmet of salvation and the sword of the Spirit, which is the word of God (Eph. 6:10, 13–17).

It is sobering to face the reality that we have to battle daily against our own destructive thoughts, emotions, and addictive behaviors; that our old nature, controlled by past experiences and past responses may reemerge time and time again. But recognizing and confessing our weaknesses and inadequacies provides for the powerful infusion of Christ's strength.

Belt of Truth

Buckle on this first piece of God's armor that holds everything else in place. First, affirm who you are by creation and by redemption. You are made in God's image; you are valuable, beloved, and pleasing to him. You are accepted by God *as you are,* and your security and significance are met in your relationship with Christ Jesus. When your self-image is securely based on God's image of you, your outer image will reflect this. Under those grave clothes is the person God designed you to be, and he wants his image of you to be seen by the world around you.

"After I participated in my first Thin Within workshop," Jane told us, "I would walk across campus wearing my voluminous purple skirt, my thighs rubbing together under its folds, saying, 'I am melting down to the size God designed me to be.' Every day I would say to myself, 'My body is not my own; it was bought at a price. I am melting down to the size God designed me to be.' God promises that 'whatever exists has already been named, and what man is has been known' (Eccles. 6:10). As I followed the Thin Within principles, the weight began to slip away, and today, five sizes smaller, I have accepted and cherish God's design for my body. That is a miracle."

When we know and apply God's truth in our lives, we affirm the truth and conform to our new identity in Christ. We live in the light, allowing no shadow of denial or deceit to obscure our honesty and integrity. We walk girded with truth, and our attitude toward our addiction, ourselves, and others is bathed in that light.

Breastplate of Righteousness

Go forward with the breastplate of righteousness in place. Righteousness is a gift; we cannot earn it nor can we manufacture it. Righteousness begins with our justification in Christ and continues as we live new lives in the Spirit, making new choices, responding reflectively and authentically in present time.

Jane continues, "After the workshops I was able to make choices that enabled me to live an empowered life. One of the Scriptures I look to when I doubt my ability to apply the principles of weight mastery is Mark 11:22–24":

> "Have faith in God," Jesus answered. "I tell you the truth, if anyone says to this mountain, 'Go, throw yourself into the sea,' and does not doubt in his heart but believes that what he says will happen, it will be done for him. Therefore I tell you, whatever you ask for in prayer, believe that you have received it, and it will be yours."

Our righteousness is secured by bands of faith, responsibility, forgiveness, confession, and recommitment—we focus on *his* correction, not *our* perfection. When we falter, we begin again, maintaining a clear conscience before God and others.

Gospel of Peace

Walk with your feet fitted with the readiness that comes from the gospel of peace. The peace of Christ rules in our hearts, quieting our warring impulses, distracting compulsions, and the demands of our addictions. We cultivate this peace by turning

away from temptation and toward God. Whenever we find ourselves challenged, on the shifting sands of peril or temptation, we
flee back to God and the rock of his Word.

"I now know that when faced with challenges," Jane reflects,
"food is never the answer. I have dealt with three deaths in my
family, two other serious illnesses, a job layoff, painful past memories, and the trauma of a bitter divorce. Through all of these
things my weight has fluctuated no more than five pounds. That
is a true miracle that I attribute to the spiritual armor of God."

Shield of Faith

Our protection from the "all the flaming arrows of the evil one"
(Eph. 6:16) is assured by the shield of faith. These may be old
thoughts and untruths, unworkable beliefs, conditioned responses,
doubts, fears, and discouragement. They may take the form of compulsive thoughts or destructive behaviors that lead us right back
into our addictive patterns. We can raise the shield of faith against
such assaults and prevent their penetration of our being.

"I used to think it would be impossible to release weight," says
Jane, "but now look at me! I am reminded of Genesis 18:14 where
the Lord tells Sarah, who is ninety years old, that she is going to
have a baby. She laughs at God! And God says, 'Is anything too
hard for the Lord?' The answer is *no*. My faith has increased as I
realize that there is nothing that God cannot do. My God-given
size, the challenges I've been able to face, and the intimacy I experience with my Lord is testimony to that."

Helmet of Salvation

Our deliverance from sin is symbolized by the helmet of salvation. We place this on our heads and remember that no matter
how many times we fall in this struggle with food, eating, and
weight, our deliverance is assured. God lifts us up time and time
again as we turn back toward him, yearning to correct our behavior and allowing him to remove our sin. The helmet is a covering
for our heads, and it makes us conscious every moment of filling
our minds with all that is good, acceptable, and perfect, rather
than with our old, negative thoughts and beliefs.

"I kept coming back to the workshop for a deeper understanding of my compulsive behaviors," says Jane. "The principles are totally different than my diet mentality, but I believed and trusted that this was the way of life for which I yearned. I also made a choice to make a renewed effort to rebuild my spiritual life—I recommitted myself to Christ and came to a deeper understanding of God and a renewed faith in the work he wants to do through me."

Sword of the Spirit

We are to take up the sword of the Spirit, which is the Word of God. We can truly fend off the assaults of our addictions and satisfy the gnawing of our silent hunger by filling our souls with the Word of God. When you are in turmoil, faced with emotions you feel you must suppress, when you are tempted to stifle the silent hunger with food, the Word of God can satisfy you with spiritual food. "But here is the bread that comes down from heaven, which a man may eat and not die. I am the living bread that came down from heaven" (John 6:50–51).

Jane reflects, "This year I bought the New Testament on tape. It nurtures my soul. I can be fulfilled on the Word and not on food. I'm not clamoring as in the past to gratify my physical appetite because now my spiritual hunger is being satisfied."

Life for all of us is a spiritual battle. We don't want to feel the pain or the hunger or the hurt. We don't want to be vulnerable for fear of rejection. We don't want to feel our silent hunger, our desire for intimacy, because of the pain we've experienced when we've reached for it in the past. We wrap up in our grave clothes thinking we can avoid the battle—thinking we can ward off our needs on our own. We think that we can win the battle by numbing the pain, feeding the hunger, or counterfeiting intimacy in our own way. The armor of God allows us the transparency and vulnerability required to feel the pain, to let him feed the hunger, to find genuine intimacy God's way.

When we are assaulted and tempted to give way to despair and old patterns of thinking and behaving, we must remind ourselves that God has provided us the spiritual armor for holy action. We must remember that he is the ultimate source of our help and the only permanent satisfaction for our silent hunger. By comparison, our inclination to derive satisfaction from other measures turns to dust on our tongues. When we are willing to disengage from our disordered eating and have our grave clothes unwrapped layer by layer, we can engage in holy action and discover that God turns our adversity into the pathway to deliverance, spiritual growth, and delight in him.

Present-Time Eating, Present-Time Living

As we live intimately in God's presence, cultivating a daily relationship of trust and surrender to him, we open ourselves to the steady influence of his love and grow to rely consistently on that love. As we surrender more completely to the Holy Spirit, he will guide, motivate, convict, and conform us from within. As we choose, in present time, to act on the basis of our new identity, we will experience the joys of genuine intimacy with ourselves, others, and God. Surrendering to him, protected by his armor, we will find that we can delight in present-time eating and present-time living—life as he intended.

When we accept who we are in Christ, knowing that we are totally acceptable to him *just as we are,* we can begin to delight in being the person God designed us to be. Then we are freed from comparing ourselves to others and obsessing about our appearance. We are free to experience and enjoy genuine intimacy with others in present time.

The more completely we discard the idea that we are worthless and unacceptable, the more fully we can accept the truth that God loves and delights in us. That doesn't mean that he gives us everything we want; it means that he fills our hearts with the capacity to delight in him and in the people around us. As the self-consciousness and obsession with our appearance diminishes, our delight intensifies. No longer demanding that the people around us satisfy our silent hunger, no longer trapped in the notion that we have to prove our worth to them, we receive a new freedom to *be* in the present, the result being that our capacity for intimacy and our freedom to delight is greatly increased.

When we live delighting in the Lord, we begin to discover that we are developing discipline. Discipline is part of our dignity and is an important part of taking responsibility for our lives. There is a great sense of freedom in discipline. We may tend to think of discipline as a negative force, inhibiting or controlling us. Discipline, however, doesn't take away our freedom, it gives us more freedom. Rather than being controlled by externals, as when we presented our members to sin, we are guided by internals—the work of the Holy Spirit (see Romans 6:13). This internal guidance is expansive and results in more and more freedom from bondage to our old ways of thinking and behaving.

Discipline has nothing to do with fighting to gain control through willpower. That is what we try to do with legalistic diets. Discipline frees us from ensnaring obsessions and legalistic attempts to control our habitual responses, permitting us to unwrap the next layer of our grave clothes and move closer to the intimacy and holiness that we desire. "You have made known to me the path of life; you will fill me with joy in your presence, with eternal pleasures at your right hand" (Ps. 16:11).

Do you see how holy action works? It turns the world upside down. Rather than constraining us from without by some system or structure, holy action promotes responsible human freedom and increases our capacity for intimacy, delight, and the fulfillment of God's will from within. When we were bound in the grave clothes of compulsive and addictive behaviors, we lived and ate in the past, thinking we were satisfying our silent hunger with food. Our self-sufficiency deceived us into thinking that surrender, responsibility, and discipline were contrary to pleasure, delight, and love. In fact, we were impoverished by the ungodly extremes of our lives—deprived of our hearts' desires. We were attempting to use food to fill up that still, silent place that can only be filled by our living God.

As we continue to allow our grave clothes to be replaced with spiritual armor, we find God in the profound silence within. Now the silence of our silent hunger becomes a sanctified silence, an expectant silence, a silence wherein we allow God to speak to our souls. "My soul, wait only upon God and silently [surrender] to Him, for my hope and expectation are from Him" (Ps. 62:5 AMP).

Questions

1. What is holy action?
2. What does holy action include?
3. Describe each of the eight aspects of holy action.
4. What do you think life would be like for you without your grave clothes?
5. What is your spiritual armor? Write about each part of your armor and its purpose.
6. What is present-time living? What is present-time eating?
7. What is discipline, and how does it affect your life?

Scripture to Read

1. Psalm 16
2. Matthew 5:33–37
*3. Romans 12:1–2
*4. 1 Corinthians 10:12–13
5. 1 Corinthians 13:1–13
6. Philippians 1:9–11
7. 2 Timothy 1:14
8. 2 Peter 1:5–9

*We suggest that you commit this Scripture to memory.

Prayer

Dear God, thank you for helping me peel away the layers of grave clothes that have kept me bound to my old unhealthy habits and attitudes. The more transparent I become, the more vulnerable I feel, the more my desire is increased to know you intimately and to savor the life with all of its challenges that you have given me. Help me to keep my focus on you and what you are working out in me moment by moment. Help me to have the courage to look beneath the surface to see those aspects of my character you wish to change. Help me to surrender unto you and allow your Holy Spirit to direct my life. Amen.

10

Holy Life

If you dare to penetrate your own silence and dare to advance without fear into the solitude of your own heart, and seek the sharing of that solitude with the lonely other who seeks God through and with you, when you will truly receive the light and capacity to understand what is beyond words and beyond explanation because it is too close to be examined: it is the ultimate union, in the depths of your own heart, of God's spirit and your own secret inmost self, so that you and he are in truth one spirit.

Thomas Merton
The Seven Storey Mountain

"Remember how the Lord your God led you all the way in the desert these forty years, to humble you and to test you in order to know what was in your heart, whether or not you would keep his commands. He humbled you, causing you to hunger and then feeding you with manna, which neither you nor your fathers had known, to teach you that man does not live on bread alone but on every word that comes from the mouth of the Lord" (Deut. 8:2–3). In our disordered eating we have gone to the end of our tether trying to live life feeding off of the false fruits of our addictive behaviors or the ways of the world. Ultimately, at the bottom of the miry pit, dispossessed, excuses and justifications failing us, we are humbled, silenced by the truth of our condition, and, as we fall to our knees, God enfolds us in his faithful arms.

"Silence is required for deep change to occur."[1] We previously avoided this silent place because we have been afraid to experience the stillness. But it is only when we find ourselves silenced by the gravity of our condition that we can begin to experience the healing of the Great Physician. Slowing down, practicing the principles, and stopping our addictive behaviors we come into the place where we can meet our living God. Here, in the silence, God shows us what is in our hearts and speaks his response. In the silence we are stunned by what we hear. Not fury, not condemnation, but God's voice declaring his love, compassion, mercy, and grace, and his promise to make us whole.

This is the word that fills the silence: the word of love declaring that the intimacy we have sought in food, in worldly relationships, in all of our addictions, is satisfied once and for all in our relationship with Christ. Our longing for oneness, for wholeness, for completion, is brought to fulfillment "that they may be one as we are one: I in them and you in me. May they be brought to complete unity" (John 17:22–23). God is feeding us with manna that neither we nor our fathers had known.

There, in the silence, all "self-centered maneuvering"[2] is put to rest. Remembering and forgiving, we put our painful past behind us as we are brought into the blazing light of God's glory. "Wait till the Lord comes. He will bring to light what is hidden in darkness and will expose the motives of men's hearts. At that time each will receive his praise from God" (1 Cor. 4:5). Now recognizing that our compulsive behavior could never satisfy our true longing, at last, we accept manna—the true bread of life.

Jane reflects, "When I think about living a life free of my disordered eating, I think about the idea of 'first love.' When I was addicted, food was my first love. Ever since I was a child, when the going got rough, I turned to food. Food was my friend, my comforter, it was always available, and I could always turn to it for company. It has been a long process and parts of it have been painful and frightening. When I started, I didn't know what was underneath all the weight I was carrying. Through God's grace deep festering wounds were revealed, but never before I was ready to see them. They were revealed at a time when I could deal with the truth and not gain back the weight I had released. Facing and resolving my hidden past and having released more than sixty pounds, I am free from my addiction to food. I am now open to the wonder of being nourished in my whole being. My first love is God, and that love shines in the fulfillment of my dreams, in the new shape of my body, and in the intimacy I have with God, myself, and other people."

Savor Food, Savor Life

"Go and enjoy choice food and sweet drinks . . . for the joy of the Lord is your strength" (Neh. 8:10). We break our addictive patterns when, in humble dependence on God, we adopt an entirely new approach to food, eating, weight, and life itself! Our new approach is based on a solid sense of our worth in Christ. We can then fill our lives with good things—good foods, intimate relationships, fulfilling careers—things that delight and satisfy us on all levels: body, mind, and soul.

There is no peace when we are living in bondage to the things of this world. We are constantly thrashing about in a flurry of activity trying somehow to survive. We cannot be still long enough to hear the voice of our silent hunger, much less the voice of our living God. In order to savor life we must experience stillness—a stillness in our inner being; a stillness in our approach to life; a stillness in our relationship with food, eating, and weight; a stillness that will lead to an intimate relationship with God.

The principles encourage this kind of stillness. In order to eat only when your body is hungry, you must be still enough to hear your body signal true physiological hunger. When you reduce the number of distractions in order to eat in a calm environment, you will create an external environment that reflects and promotes inner stillness. When you eat only when you are sitting, you will reinforce a slow, still pace and make it possible to savor your food. By eating only when your body and mind are relaxed, you will promote a stillness and appreciation for a wonderful God-given activity—eating. When you are still and can listen for the Holy Spirit, you will begin eating only the foods you enjoy, those foods that nurture you, and you will know when to stop. In this stillness, you will savor food as never before.

As we slow down and savor our food, we will slow down and savor life itself. When we were slaves to unworkable beliefs and habitual responses, our addictive relationship to food and also to life, was unrewarding and unsatisfying. Releasing the things that no longer serve us—our fat machinery, our painful past experiences, our denial, our unforgiveness, our rebellion, the radical extremes of our eating habits, our frenetic pace—we also release the weight that burdened us for so many years. Living by grace and freedom in Christ, from a renewed mind, in the power of the Holy Spirit, we discard our mindless habits and live in the light, fully cognizant of life, reflective in our responses, satisfied by our activities, and graciously giving God the glory. Living by grace with freedom in Christ means that with the power of the Holy Spirit we are no longer under the control of our feelings, cravings, and urges, but we can live according to the conscious choices we make in obedience to his will.

When I (Judy) was bulimic, I would frequently say that the reason I ate too much was that I just *loved* food. My rationale was totally false. The reason I was eating too much was that it was a compulsion, an addiction. I had taken it out of God's hands and into my own hands. I didn't love food; I lusted after it. When we are in our addictions, we love nothing. We have to quiet down to love; we have to become still to savor food, to savor life!

In this stillness we experience our hunger for God, and then he feeds us with manna. The bread of heaven is a symbol of our dependence on God for just what we need to nourish us day by day. This heavenly food is precisely the opposite of our addictive food—we cannot create it ourselves, and we cannot hoard it to eat compulsively; we must rely on God to give it to us moment by moment according to our needs. The principles encourage stillness and our ability to wait on God to feed us and lead us. This cannot happen as we're standing up stuffing food into our mouths, or devouring our fast-food fix as we're driving down the freeway.

This can happen only as we wait, in the stillness, for that which comes only from the Father's hand.

God Satisfies Our Deepest Hunger

We are created for relationship and intimacy and for the profound sense of security, significance, and self-worth that comes out of being truly loved and cherished. Our longing for intimacy, for that astounding relationship that embraces us, body, mind, and soul, is so profound that when it is lacking we may take matters into our own hands and devise strategies in an attempt to find some relief or satisfaction, as the following story illustrates.

In 1981 the new disease AIDS was reported. It exploded into an epidemic. As part of my (Arthur's) medical practice, I volunteered one day a week to work in an AIDS clinic in San Francisco. Over the next six years I watched several hundred young men die of this disease. One patient, a very bright young man named Mark, told me that he used to frequent the gay bath houses and would often have sex with as many as a dozen men a night, many of whose names he didn't even know. Deeply grieved, I asked Mark why he had put himself at such risk. His answer was very simple, "Dr. Halliday, I was looking for love."

I was shocked by this remark. I was not a Christian at the time, and I had very little understanding of what Mark meant. I realized that even though I was Mark's doctor and was supposed to be caring for his needs, I didn't know how to give him what he was searching for. Mark died shortly thereafter without finding that love.

Not only did this experience communicate the tragic emptiness and self-destruction that comes into our lives when we desperately attempt to replace our legitimate silent hunger with counterfeit intimacy, but it also had a profound effect on me personally. About two weeks later, at 1:38 A.M. on June 25, 1984, I awakened from a sound sleep and felt engulfed by the most profound love I had ever experienced. I didn't see or hear anything. I didn't say anything. But I realized that what I was experiencing was the love of Jesus Christ. This demonstrated to me that Jesus is who he said he is, that his existence is real, and that he was to be my salvation. I gave my life to the Lord at that moment.

When we turn to God and are willing to allow our grave clothes to be unwrapped, the Holy Spirit will begin the healing process. We will find ourselves mightily blessed when we allow him to lead us from our darkness into his light. Our painful past is a significant part of this process, because, having experienced misery firsthand, we appreciate and can share with others much more fully the beauty, peace, joy, and love that come from God's healing hand. Because of where we have been, we can more deeply appreciate the wonder, beauty, and joy of where we are now.

Genuine Intimacy

"I recently visited my father for the first time in twenty-eight years. I was ready to take this risk because I felt free enough from the hurts of the past. After a warm greeting, with tears in his eyes, he said, 'Hannah, I'm so sorry I wasn't around to see you grow up.' He spoke of how sad he had been, thinking of me with no daddy, and acknowledged that he had lost out as well, especially all the years of intimacy we might have had. The amazing thing was that I felt no bitterness in my heart—just compassion for both of us. I had changed and matured to the point of being able to accept the situation and his love for me with deep gratitude. One of the lessons I learned concerns receiving love. I must let people love me in their own way and in their own time. I now feel comfortable with myself for the first time. All the years of healing, risking, trusting, and changing, as painful as they were, have been a blessing. In the process I have released seventy pounds. There is more work to be done, but the more intimate I become with God, the better it gets."

Much about disordered eating is based on our inability to receive love, even more than our inability to give it. We often manipulate the people in our lives to give us what we didn't get. As we are healed by God's love, we are then able to accept love from others, freed from our expectations and demands that love come when we want it, in the exact form we want it, and from whom we want it.

Maybe we feel ashamed or unworthy, or maybe we are still too bitter or too demanding. It is not always the case that love isn't there; often it is. Those grave clothes block not only our ability to give love but to receive it.

Because in the past we've missed the love we've wanted, we're afraid of being vulnerable for fear of being hurt again. The fear of disappointment is so profound and the silent hunger is so acute that we will attempt to feed it with our addictions rather than risk exposing ourselves. By unwrapping our grave clothes, we reveal our true hunger, and the Holy Spirit moves in our lives and relationships so that we are fed.

> *By eating what God directs us to eat, we rediscover the delights of good food and experience the joy of being the size God designed us to be.*

Our healing involves far more than just a resolution of our issues with food, eating, and weight. By allowing God to fulfill our inborn desire for intimacy and satisfy our need for security, significance, and self-worth, we can, in turn, glorify him in body, mind, and soul. When we began this process, we committed ourselves to deal with the attitudes, habits, and eating patterns that had accumulated as we tried unsuccessfully on our own to stifle the voice of our silent hunger. Little did we know how profoundly God wished to transform our character during our healing or how unsurpassed would be the delights he had in store for us. By replacing the grave clothes of our past with the spiritual armor of God in the present, we have established a new relationship with food, eating, and our bodies. By eating what God directs us to eat, we rediscover the delights of good food and experience the joy of being the size God designed us to be. No longer attempting to satisfy our inner longings with food, we sweep our house clean, leaving room for God to meet our deepest need for intimacy in relationship. Once our silent hunger is satisfied, our purpose can be redirected from self-centered attempts to gratify ourselves to a selfless sacrifice for others. "True spirituality moves beyond self-actualization to the consideration of others."[3]

This, then, is our healing process: God leads us out of the darkness of our disordered eating to honesty and repentance about the past, through forgiving others and being forgiven ourselves, to a knowledge and experience of God's love. Receiving security and significance out of our true identity as children of a good and loving Father by way of Christ's death on our behalf, we can cast aside our old unworkable beliefs, past experiences, conditioned and habitual responses. We put on spiritual armor and, in freedom to be vulnerable and authentic, we are given the courage and strength to approach others, establishing trust, intimacy, and loving relationships. Herein lies the satisfaction of our silent hunger—true intimacy with God, with ourselves, and with others.

Genuine intimacy allows us to receive his love and the love of others. It frees us to love God openly and expressively and to minister to others with self-giving love. Intimacy keeps us calmly in the silence. Through intimacy, God is glorified in relationship. Intimacy allows us to have an abundant life that shines, a life that glorifies, a life that is able to receive the love that God has provided.

> ## *The most satisfied and delighted we will ever be is when we glorify God.*

The ability to experience this intimacy and to delight in the fullness of our life on earth in the present prepares us to enter with eagerness into the heavenly places when he calls. It is part of the sanctification process that we experience satisfaction and joy every step of the way. "The enjoyment of God and the glorification of God are one. His eternal purpose and our eternal pleasure unite. The chief end of man is to glorify God by enjoying Him forever."[4] The most satisfied and delighted we will ever be is when we glorify God. Having begun the unwrapping, having experienced satisfaction and delight, we have the assurance that "he who began a good work in you will carry it on to completion until the day of Christ" (Phil. 1:6).

Questions

1. What is a holy life?
2. How do we savor life?
3. How do the Thin Within principles encourage stillness?
4. What is genuine intimacy?
5. What is the purpose of allowing our grave clothes to be removed?
6. How are the enjoyment of God and the glorification of God one?
7. In what ways do you see God completing a good work in you right now?

Scripture to Read

1. Deuteronomy 8:2–3
2. Nehemiah 8:10
3. Psalm 51
4. John 17:20–26
5. 1 Corinthians 4:1–4
*6. Philippians 1:6

*We suggest that you commit this Scripture to memory.

Prayer

Dear God, thank you that you have provided a way for me to live a holy life—not a perfect life but a life that allows me to come to you humbly just as I am. In the still silence of our intimacy, help me to listen for your voice as you instruct me and teach me. I pray that you will help me to set aside quiet time to be sensitive to your leading, as you continue to peel away the layers of my self-centered behavior. I pray that you will help me not to hold back from an intimate loving relationship with you, and that I will allow you to use me to reach out in love to others who are hurting. Help me to let your light shine before many that they may see your good deeds and praise you! Thank you. Amen.

Additional Resources

Reconciling with
Your Body

Those of us who struggle with issues of food, eating, and weight have a tendency to hate our bodies. We manifest, whether through overeating or other compulsive behaviors, the belief, derived from our limited or distorted experience of intimacy, that we are irredeemably flawed. We condemn our bodies for betraying us by repeatedly seeking gratification from food. We condemn our bodies for lacking the self-control that would insure permanent weight loss. We condemn our bodies for not looking perfect, for not *being* perfect. Our weight thus becomes both the arena in which we play out our negative self-image and the reason for our self-hatred. As a result, we lose the ability to distinguish between our weight and our person—we forget who we really are in Christ. We loathe our bodies because they don't fit some preconceived idealized image, so we violate them, and, in the end, we lose our ability to appreciate that our bodies are "fearfully [lovingly] and wonderfully made" (Ps. 139:14a).

Obsessed with hating and condemning our bodies, we reflect our fundamental inability to accept ourselves for who we really are. John Stott, in *The Cross of Christ,* writes, "My true self is what I am by creation, which Christ came to redeem, and by calling."[1] In this, our true self, abides our dignity and the basis for our self-acceptance. The good news is that we can develop a secure and loving sense of ourselves based on God's knowledge of us. When our dignity and self-acceptance rest in our appearance, we can become discouraged and depressed, and we eat, drink, and despair. But if we can accept the fact that God sees us as worthy enough for the sacrifice of his son, we suddenly discover that there is nothing to condemn. "Therefore, there is now no condemnation for those who are in Christ Jesus, because through Christ Jesus the law of the Spirit of life set me free from the law of sin and death" (Rom. 8:1–2).

In God's presence you can begin to experience within your body and mind the creation God intended you to be, giving voice to your silent hunger and releasing your excess weight. The important thing to realize is that satisfaction with your body comes when you take your assessment from God, not from magazines, TV, or your mirror! Accepting this truth and not being intimidated by Hollywood or Madison Avenue requires a strong sense of security and significance. You have a God-given size and shape that are uniquely yours, and God invites you to discover, establish, and celebrate your complexity and to accept your new image based on his unique design for you. "[Y]our works are wonderful, I know that full well. My frame was not hidden from you when I was made in the secret place. When I was woven together in the depth of the earth, your eyes saw my unformed body" (Ps. 139:14b–15).

Our faith in God's Word affirms the goodness of the body. We know that God created us in his image and pronounced his creation good. "God saw all that he had made, and it was very good" (Gen. 1:31). We know, beyond that, that God was pleased with creation: "thou hast created all things, and for thy pleasure they are and were created" (Rev. 4:11). We know that God chose to enter our world in the flesh. He lived, ate, drank, laughed, cried, and died as one of us—in a body. "The Word became flesh and made his dwelling among us" (John 1:14), "for in Christ all the fullness of the Deity lives in bodily form" (Col. 2:9). Furthermore, Christ gave his body for us in his death on the cross, and gives it to us symbolically time and again in the sacrament of holy communion: "This is my body given for you" (Luke 22:19). And God is not done with our bodies, even after death. "The body that is sown is perishable, it is raised imperishable. . . . [I]t is sown a natural body, it is raised a spiritual body" (1 Cor. 15:42–44). Finally, we know that our bodies are of such surpassing good that God's Spirit has chosen to reside in us. "Don't you know that you yourselves are God's temple and that God's Spirit lives in you?" (1 Cor. 3:16). Your body is precious to God. It is a magnificent creation intended to be cared for and cherished, "therefore, honor God with your body" (1 Cor. 7:4).

The Body Exercise that follows will allow you to begin a conversation with your body. In this exercise we silence all negative or critical thoughts about ourselves and begin to honor our bodies. We encourage you to be compassionate toward *all* parts of your body, especially those parts you have disliked the most. You will begin to use language that is filled with acceptance, not anger or condemnation, language that is appreciative. As you do, you will begin to see that your body is a miraculous creation, worthy to be acknowledged as the glorious gift that it is.

The Body Awareness Exercise

The following exercise will give you a new perspective on your body and an increased appreciation for the marvelous gift it is.

Stand with your feet about one foot apart. Mark sure you feel stable, so you will be comfortable with your eyes closed. Let your arms hang freely at your sides and close your eyes. Be aware of your breathing, the rise and fall of your chest as the breath comes in and out. Now focus on your body—if there are areas in which you feel uncomfortable or tense, see if you can relax and loosen up a bit.

Now, start with your feet. Be aware of your feet, noticing which part of your feet supports your weight. How do you feel about your feet? How have they served you over the years? Take a moment and express your gratitude for your feet.

Now become aware of your calves. What sensations do you have in your calves? What thoughts and feelings do you have about your calves? How have they served you? Take a moment and express your appreciation for your calves.

Now focus your attention on your knees. What sensations do you experience in your knees? What thoughts and feelings do you have about your knees? How have they served you? Take a moment and express your appreciation for your knees.

Now become aware of your upper legs. What thoughts and feelings do you have about your upper legs? Take your hands and feel the front and back of your upper legs. Notice the size and shape of your legs. Do they feel the same as, better than, or worse than you thought they would? How have your upper legs served you? Take a moment and express your gratitude for your upper legs.

194

Now become aware of your hips and buttocks. What sensations do you have in this area? What thoughts and feelings do you have about your hips and buttocks? With your hands notice how the entire area feels. Does it feel the way you thought it would? How have your hips and buttocks served you? Take a moment and express your appreciation for your hips and buttocks.

Now become aware of your stomach and abdomen. What sensations do you have in the area of your stomach and abdomen? What thoughts and feelings do you have about your stomach and abdomen? Take a moment and feel your stomach and abdomen. Do you feel full or hungry right now? How has your stomach served you? Take a moment and express your gratitude.

Now become aware of your chest and rib cage. What sensations do you have in this area? Take a moment and feel your chest and rib cage. What thoughts and feelings do you have about your chest and rib cage? How have they served you? Take a moment and express your appreciation for your chest and rib cage.

Let your arms hang down by your sides. How do you feel about your arms? What thoughts and feelings do you have about your arms? Feel your upper and lower arms with your hands. How have they served you over the years? Take a moment and express your gratitude for your arms and hands.

Become aware of your shoulders and the area between your shoulder blades. Is this area tight, uncomfortable, or stiff? If so, move your shoulders around; raise and lower them to loosen them up a bit. Do the same with your neck—roll your head around, first one way, then the other. Take a moment and express your appreciation for your shoulders and upper back.

Now focus your attention on your face. What sensations do you have in your face? Slowly feel your face and notice how it feels. Feel the area under your chin, your neck, your hair. How has your face served you? Take a moment and express your appreciation for your face.

Now consider that God has created your unique body—you are his creation, his workmanship, even if in some ways you appear different than you desire. Thank the Lord for the unique body that he has given you.

Medical Issues and Family Eating Patterns

Arthur Halliday, M.D.

The spectrum of eating disorders ranges from those whose obesity or anorexia is life-threatening to those whose lives are controlled or dictated by food and eating because of their obsession with their appearance. This includes millions of people who suffer because they have a disordered relationship with food. The physical, psychological, emotional, and spiritual suffering from these problems is incalculable, and unfortunately the problem seems to be getting worse, as evidenced by the following statistics:

- 44 percent of high school girls and 15 percent of high school boys reported they were trying to lose weight.[1]
- 1 in 3 Americans is estimated to be overweight, an increase of 30 percent in the past ten years.[2]
- 50 percent of adult females and 24 percent of adult males are on a diet at any given time.[3]
- Close to 80 percent of pre-pubescent girls, some as young as eight or nine, restrict their eating for fear of getting fat.[4]
- It was estimated in 1982 that 1 in 250 adolescent females was anorexic or bulimic. The incidence is clearly much higher now.[5]
- It is estimated that 10 percent of Americans have disordered eating, 20 percent of those in college.[6]

196

While it is well established that the root causes of these disorders are complex, it is our firm belief that:

1. A person's excess weight and/or disordered eating are always *symptoms* of an underlying problem or false belief, and that permanent resolution depends on identifying and correcting the cause, whether it be physical, emotional, or spiritual.
2. The vast majority of these problems are spiritual in origin and therefore require spiritual solutions.
3. Therapy limited to changing one's weight or eating habits by external means (diets, shots, pills, exercise) rarely succeeds.

Since disordered eating usually has its origins in the formative years, and since an ounce of prevention is always worth more than a pound of cure, it is worthwhile to look at children and eating. A detailed discussion of this subject is beyond the scope of this book, so interested readers are referred to the suggested readings at the end of this section, from which the following are excerpts:

- Putting a child on a diet is the worst thing a person can do, where food is concerned.
- Withholding food can make a youngster feel very unhappy about him- or herself. An overweight child's self-esteem is already under siege by the taunts of other children and the comments of insensitive adults, but it's the parents' approval that is the most important—the child wants to please them more than anything else. If they ration food, it will confirm the child's fear that something is wrong with him or her. The child will feel that he or she has failed by wanting to eat more than the parents want to give.
- Parents may think it is their duty to make their overweight child "thin" no matter what, but they must avoid the temptation to put him or her on a diet. It simply will not work, because a youngster will usually find a way to eat the "forbidden" foods, if not at home then at a friend's house. Because of the child's determination to eat what he or she wants, the diet is doomed from the start.

- Any scheme to get a child to lose weight via a diet is worse than useless—it's damaging. That's because it can make an overweight child even more preoccupied with food than before, and therefore more apt to overeat whenever possible. Excess weight (particularly in girls) was highly associated with the degree to which the parents tried to restrain their children's eating.
- Putting children on diets presupposes that their excess weight is their own fault due to a lack of willpower, self-control, or motivation. Nothing could be further from the truth, since eating disorders have a variety of causes, many of which children probably don't understand or over which they have no control.
- Today's children are much less physically active and therefore burn many fewer calories than the children of previous generations. They often watch as much as twenty-four hours of TV per week.
- Eating disorders in children are often a sign of something amiss in the family dynamics. It may come from a child's loneliness, pain, anger, or as a surrogate for intimacy that is lacking between parents and children. Parents who find it hard to give their children close, loving support may try to compensate by overfeeding or allowing the children to overfeed themselves. In other cases children may medicate or sedate themselves with food in order to make it easier to deal with lack of acceptance, family strife, or a disruption, such as death or divorce. Eating disorders may become a family's "symptom of choice" for unresolved issues that have nothing otherwise to do with food.
- Here are some basic steps all parents can take, no matter what the reason for a child's eating problem:
  1. Just be concerned with overall good health and nutrition, making healthy choices available, and leave it at that. There is no need to focus on *how much* the child eats. Each of us is born with a finely tuned internal mechanism (our hunger scale) for regulating the amount of food we need to eat. This is a reliable system, particularly in children, unless it is overridden by some

outside interference. Even overweight children should be allowed to decide how much to eat. If allowed to regulate their own intake (with no external pressure), after a few weeks children will begin to "hear" their own inner signals of hunger and satiety and will eat less as a result. They will develop discipline from within.

2. All children should be subject to *regular* meals and snack times, and the food served at the appointed times should generally be nutritious selections of the parents' choice. Allowing children (if they are old enough) to have some voice in the selection and preparation of foods can create a feeling of teamwork as well as mutual trust. For example, each child might be allowed to select one item he or she enjoys to be served at a specific meal.

3. Parents need to learn to trust their children's instincts, leave them free of emotional discomfort caused by outside interference, and acknowledge their biological right to decide how much they eat. Eating disorders expert Hilde Bruch found that children who have the least treatment for their obesity are the most likely to resolve their weight problems later in life.

- Success cannot be measured on the scales. Some children's bodies simply are not meant to turn out as slender as their parents would like. This is not easy to accept when parents have the brightest hopes for their children, wanting them to be perfect. But it's important for them to know that it's okay if the child does not meet the societal image of perfection. The important thing is that they be the size God intended them to be.

- What is more important than their weight is that children grow up to be adults who like themselves. For parents this means allowing their children to grow up emotionally, physically, and spiritually healthy by offering the love and instilling the confidence that a child must have as a foundation for a full and rewarding life. Children must know that they are loved and accepted as they are and that it has nothing to do with their weight.

- Parents can turn off the TV and tell children it's up to them to figure out something to do. Boredom arising from a turned-off TV generates self-reliance and creativity. It's perfectly reasonable to send children outside to play and in that way to encourage "vigorous fun."
- Emotionally *unhealthy* overweight adults often come from households in which their parents were preoccupied with their child's excess weight and tried to get rid of it. Emotionally *healthy* overweight adults, on the other hand, were generally raised by parents who didn't define their children by their weight. Instead, the parents approved of their children and were proud of them for who they were and were not dissatisfied because their children didn't "measure up."

Suggested Readings

Reiff, Dan W., M.P.H., R.D., and Kathleen Kim Lampson Reiff, Ph.D., *Eating Disorders: Nutrition Therapy in the Recovery Process*, Aspen Publishers, Gaithersburg, MD, 1992.

Satter, Ellyn, *How to Get Your Child to Eat . . . But Not Too Much*, Bull Publishers, Palo Alto, CA, 1992.

"Tufts University Diet and Nutrition Letter," Vol. 11, No. 10, December 1993.

Medical Questions Frequently Asked at Thin Within Workshops

Arthur Halliday, M.D.

Q: Won't I develop low blood sugar if I wait too long to eat? If I skip a meal I tend to get nervous and shaky.

A: Symptomatic hypoglycemia (low blood sugar) does occur, but contrary to the reports in the lay press, it is rather rare. To establish this diagnosis you must have (1) legitimate symptoms, (2) a documented low blood sugar at the time there are symptoms, and (3) prompt relief within five or ten minutes after eating. Most often such symptoms are due to some other cause.

Q: You say there are no forbidden foods, but what about cholesterol? And aren't there other medical conditions where certain foods are prohibited?

A: It is always important to check with your physician to be sure there are no dietary restrictions (such as diabetes, some diseases of the liver and kidneys, and high cholesterol situations). Our experience is that as people practice the Thin Within principles they begin to choose healthier foods, and as they release weight, their cholesterol levels usually drop. Naturally, we always recommend that people keep their fat intake at approximately thirty grams or less per day. This is not a rigid rule, and we don't recommend counting grams of fat, which can become another legalistic system. We say if you want to release fat, continue to decrease fat.

Q: Is it necessary to take vitamins, minerals, or food supplements while releasing weight?

A: As long as your food intake is well-balanced, it shouldn't be necessary. I personally think Americans spend far too much money on such products—that getting them naturally through our food is best. If you feel you must take vitamins, I would limit it to a one-a-day multiple vitamin.

Q: Can I practice the Thin Within principles during pregnancy?

A: Absolutely—but be sure to tell your obstetrician what you are doing. And you will need to take extra vitamin/mineral supplements.

Q: Will my set point change if I try to "lose" weight?

A: This is a controversial subject. There is data that shows that as we radically decrease our food intake our metabolic rate (so-called "set point") decreases, making it more difficult to release weight, but our experience is that if you release weight slowly this isn't a problem.

Q: I tend to eat compulsively during my premenstrual period. What should I do?

A: This is a fairly common complaint, and you should check with your physician to see if there is a medical explanation for your cravings. In any event, following the principles is the best solution for compulsive eating no matter when it occurs.

Q: Is it necessary to eat three meals a day?

A: Not unless your work is physically very demanding. Many people do fine eating only once or twice a day. Don't forget, you can trust your body to indicate when or how often it is time to eat. If you choose to eat more frequently, you will find that a light snack (eating "0" to "3") will allow you to get to your "0" more often. This is an acceptable option for those who prefer to eat more frequently.

Q: Can children follow the principles?

A: Yes—most of them do it naturally.

Q: My children want to eat only "junk" food. Should I let them?

A: Studies have consistently shown that if you continue to offer kids predominantly healthy foods (and don't fuss too much about the "junk"), they will gradually incorporate more nutritious foods into their diets.

Q: How rapidly can I lose weight without upsetting my metabolism?

A: I tell people one pound per week—determined by what your clothes and the mirror tell you, not by your scale! It should be fairly easy to do this and have a good, balanced intake of foods you enjoy. At this rate, you won't lose your skin tone (no flabby excess skin) as happens with rapid weight loss. Also, releasing weight over a longer period gives your body time to adjust to the new way of eating so that it will be second nature to you when you reach your desired weight. Most of us put weight on slowly: It seems natural to take it off at the same rate. (There are also some medical hazards—gall stones being one—of rapid weight loss.)

Q: How important is physical activity in losing weight?

A: It takes an enormous amount of exercise by itself to release a significant amount of weight. However, physical activity is very good for us, especially for the cardiovascular system, and it is an excellent adjunct for improving body tone when combined with our improved eating habits. We encourage you to exercise for at least thirty minutes three times a week, preferably doing something you enjoy. It will help you be more attuned to your body's messages.

Q: Is it normal to gain weight as we age?

A: No, but it is so common that obesity is considered the most common nutritional problem of the elderly in this country. It results from our being less physically active and yet continuing to eat as we did in our more physically active years. The simple solution is to eat less according to your body's needs and exercise more. Walking is especially good.

For further questions or comments about this information, medical or otherwise, please write us at:

Thin Within
101 First Street, #438
Los Altos, CA 94022

Notes

Chapter 1

1. Dan W. Reiff and Kathleen Kim Lampson Reiff, *Eating Disorders: Nutrition Therapy in the Recovery Process* (Gaithersburg, Md.: Aspen Publishers, 1992), 5.

2. Ibid.

3. Adapted from Reiff and Reiff, *Eating Disorders,* 5.

4. Larry Crabb, *Marriage Builder* (Grand Rapids: Zondervan Publishing Co., 1982), 19.

5. Ibid., 8.

6. These points are adapted from Reiff and Reiff, *Eating Disorders,* 8.

7. Ibid., 9.

8. Gerald G. May, *Addiction and Grace* (San Francisco: Harper & Row, 1988), 1.

Chapter 2

1. Eugene H. Peterson, *Traveling Light: Modern Meditations on St. Paul's Letter of Freedom* (Colorado Springs: Helmers & Howard, 1988), 103.

2. Ibid.

3. Marcel Proust, *Remembrance of Things Past.*

4. The grave clothes image is adapted from Keith Miller's audio tape, "The Miracle of Intimacy."

5. John Owen, *Sin & Temptation: The Challenge to Personal Godliness* (Portland, Oreg.: Multnomah Press, 1983), 36–37.

6. Brennan Manning, *The Ragamuffin Gospel: Good News for the Bedraggled, Beat-Up, and Burnt Out* (Portland, Oreg.: Multnomah, 1990), 157.

7. Brother Lawrence, *The Practice of the Presence of God* (Springdale, Pa.: Whitaker House, 1982), 51.

8. Manning, *The Ragamuffin Gospel,* 174.

9. Model adapted from "Acceptance Seminar: How God's Acceptance Can Change Our Inner Life" by David Eckman. Presented at Peninsula Bible Church, Cupertino, Calif., Fall 1993.

10. Flora Slosson Wuellner, *Prayer, Stress, and Our Inner Wounds* (Nashville: The Upper Room, 1985), 14.

11. Genesis 1:27; Romans 8:29; James 3:9.

12. John 1:12; Romans 8:16; Ephesians 1:4; 1 Peter 2:9; 1 John 3:1.

13. John 3:16–17; 1 Corinthians 6:20; 7:23.

14. Colossians 1:19–22.

15. Romans 8:17; Galatians 3:29; 4:7.

Chapter 3

1. May, *Addiction and Grace,* 120.

2. Paul Tournier, "Guilt and Grace," in *The Best of Paul Tournier* (New York: Iverson-Norman, 1977), 121. See also Romans 4:13ff.; Galatians 3:1–20.

3. Tournier, "Guilt and Grace," 121.

4. May, *Addiction and Grace,* 17.

5. Reiff and Reiff, *Eating Disorders,* 245.

6. Tournier, *Guilt and Grace,* 122.

7. Manning, *The Ragamuffin Gospel,* 214.

Chapter 4

1. Peterson, *Traveling Light,* 23.

2. Eckman, "Acceptance Seminar."

3. David Seamands, *Healing for Damaged Emotions* (Bethesda, Md.: Scripture Press Publications, 1991), 73.

4. May, *Addiction and Grace,* 150.

Chapter 5

1. Sandra D. Wilson, *Released from Shame: Recovery for Adult Children of Dysfunctional Families* (Downers Grove, Ill.: InterVarsity Press, 1990), 28.

2. Dan Allender, "Intimacy," (lecture given in San Diego, Calif., 1992).

3. Wilson, *Released from Shame,* 31.

4. Ibid.

5. Allender, "Intimacy."

6. Gershen Kaufman, *Shame: The Power of Caring* (Cambridge, Mass.: Schenkman Books, 1985), 165.

7. Stott, *Cross of Christ,* 96.

8. Bruce Narramore, *No Condemnation* (Grand Rapids: Zondervan Publishing Co., 1984), 149.

9. Ibid.

10. Manning, *The Ragamuffin Gospel,* 115.

11. Tournier, *The Best of Paul Tournier,* 117.

12. Dan Allender, *The Wounded Heart: Hope for Adult Victims of Childhood Sexual Abuse* (Colorado Springs: NavPress, 1990), 192.

13. Tournier, *The Best of Paul Tournier,* 65.

14. Albert Nolan, *Jesus Before Christianity* (Maryknoll, N.Y.: Orbis Books, 1978), 56.

15. Tournier, *The Best of Paul Tournier,* 112.

16. Peterson, *Traveling Light,* 36.

17. Robert Rosenthal and Lenore Hacobson, *Pygmalion in the Classroom: Teacher Expectation and Pupil Intellectual Development* (New York: Holt, Rinehart and Winston, 1968), 61–71.

Chapter 6

1. For a more complete discussion of *addicere* and addiction as a "quasireligious imitation of surrender to the Sacred," see Adrian van Kaam, *Fulfillment in the Spiritual Life* (Wilkes-Barre, Pa.: Personal Dimension Books, 1966), 124.

2. May, *Addiction and Grace*, 13.

3. Ibid., 40.

4. Paul Tournier, *Creative Suffering*, quoted in Stott, *Cross of Christ* (Downers Grove, Ill.: InterVarsity Press, 1986), 319 (author's emphasis).

5. May, *Addiction and Grace*, 169.

Chapter 7

1. These stages of grief are based on the work of Dr. Elisabeth Kübler-Ross. See her *On Death and Dying* (New York: Macmillan, 1969).

2. Lewis B. Smedes, *Forgive and Forget: Healing the Hurts We Don't Deserve* (San Francisco: Harper & Row, 1984), xi.

3. Joanne Ross Feldmeth and Midge Wallace Finely, *We Weep for Ourselves and Our Children: A Christian Guide for Survivors of Childhood Sexual Abuse* (San Francisco: Harper & Row, 1990), 130. See also Romans 12:17.

4. Smedes, *Forgive and Forget*, 108.

5. James D. Berkeley, "When It's Better Not to Forgive: Ethicist Lewis Smedes Goes Beyond the Cheap Apology," in *Marriage Partnership* (Winter 1991), 73.

6. Smedes, *Forgive and Forget*, 108.

7. Ibid., 38–39.

8. Ibid.

9. Ibid., 133.

10. G. P. Mellick Belshaw, ed. *Lent with Evelyn Underhill: Selections from Her Writings,* (Ridgefield, Conn.: Morehouse Publishing, 1990), 24.

11. Robert S. McGee, "The Blame Game," 5.

12. Wuellner, *Prayer, Stress, and Our Inner Wounds*, 34.

13. Ibid., 34–35.

Chapter 8

1. M. R. Vincent, *Word Studies in the New Testament* (McLean, Va.: McDonald Publishing Co., 1984), 701.

2. Ray Stedman, *From Guilt to Glory*, Vol. 1 (Portland, Oreg.: Multnomah Press, 1973), 57.

3. Adapted from Greg Burts, "Choices," a paper presented at a seminar of Christian counseling at First Baptist Church, Los Altos, Ca., Sept. 1988.

4. May, *Addiction and Grace*, 139.

5. Robert S. McGee, *The Search for Significance* (Houston: Rapha Publishing, 1988), 144.

6. John Murray, *Principles of Conduct* (Grand Rapids: Eerdmans, 1957), 38–39.

7. Ibid., 39.

Chapter 9

1. Burts, "Choices."
2. May, *Addiction and Grace,* 122.
3. Stott, *The Cross of Christ,* 96.
4. Ibid.
5. Ibid., 101.
6. John Hannemon, "Message on Prayer: Luke 11:1–13," catalog no. 926 (Cupertino, Ca.: Peninsula Bible Church, July 11, 1993).
7. Ibid.
8. Ibid.
9. Mother Teresa of Calcutta, quoted by Bill Volkman, "Our Resident Psychotherapist," in *Union Life* (May/June 1991), 10.
10. May, *Addiction and Grace,* 168.
11. Much of the following material on boundaries is adapted from the Minirth-Meier Clinic West Seminars in the topic "Boundaries: Key to Freedom, Key to Love."
12. Ibid.

Chapter 10

1. Dan Allender, *Bold Love* (Colorado Springs: NavPress, 1992), 68.
2. Ibid., 75.
3. David Allen, *In Search of the Heart* (Nashville: Thomas Nelson, 1982), 146.
4. John Piper, *Desiring God* (Portland, Oreg.: Multnomah Press, 1986), 226.

Reconciling with Your Body

1. Stott, *The Cross of Christ,* 285.

Medical Issues and Family Eating Patterns

1. Centers for Disease Control and Prevention, Atlanta, Ga.
2. Ibid.
3. *USA Today,* August 11, 1986.
4. "Dieting: The Losing Game," *Time,* January 20, 1986.
5. R. E. Kendall, et al., "The Epidemiology of Anorexia Nervosa," *Psychological Medicine,* 3 (1973).
6. Ibid.